HEALTHY BRAIN
ORIGAMI

Fold Decorative Paper Models That Boost Mental Acumen and Keep Your Brain Active!

MAYUMI OHARA AND **KATSUSHI YOKOI**

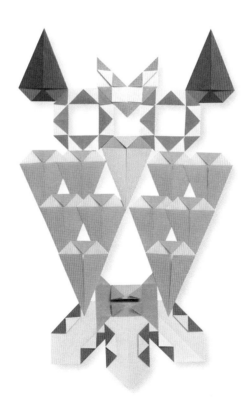

TUTTLE Publishing

Tokyo | Rutland, Vermont | Singapore

Contents

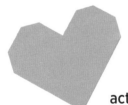

Enjoy these easy-to-follow, effective brain-training activities that keep your mind sharp with modular origami

Combine simple origami components to create colorful, kaleidoscopic paper artworks. You can use any regular origami paper that's available for purchase almost everywhere you shop. Choose your favorite colors and create your favorite pieces whenever you like.

Folding the components is easy, but assembling them into a larger artwork requires a bit of ingenuity. Carefully study the provided photos of the finished examples. From these, you can usually figure out how to make the pieces on your own. But if you get stumped, refer to the instructions provided as "methods."

From choosing the paper to thinking about how to display, use and gift your creations—these are all brain-training activities. Observe with your eyes, make decisions with your brain, coordinate the movements of your fingertips, and take actions to assemble and display your decorations. Make brain training a habit through modular origami and actively enjoy your life!

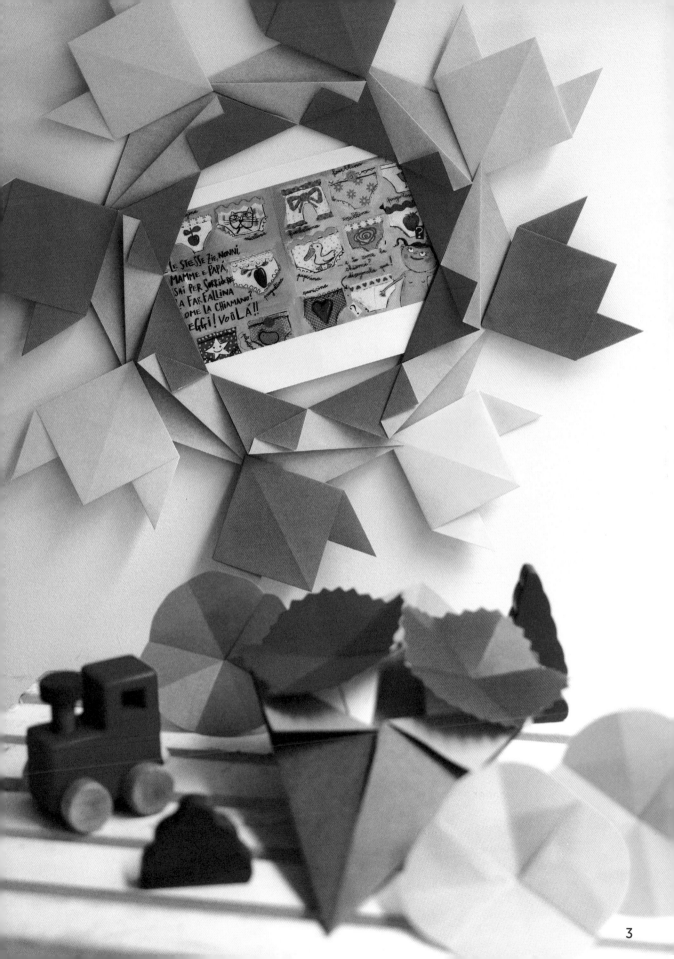

Catalog of Basic Origami Parts

24 Parts + 4 Origami Models

There are 24 basic origami parts described in this book. In addition to these basic parts, we will introduce four origami models that combine well with other designs. Remember their names and shapes, and use these pages as a quick reference.

In this book, we show photos of the finished decorations, but in fact, the different ways to combine the parts are practically unlimited. Learn the basic techniques by folding and assembling the projects in this book, and then challenge yourself to create new configurations using your own ideas for inspiration.

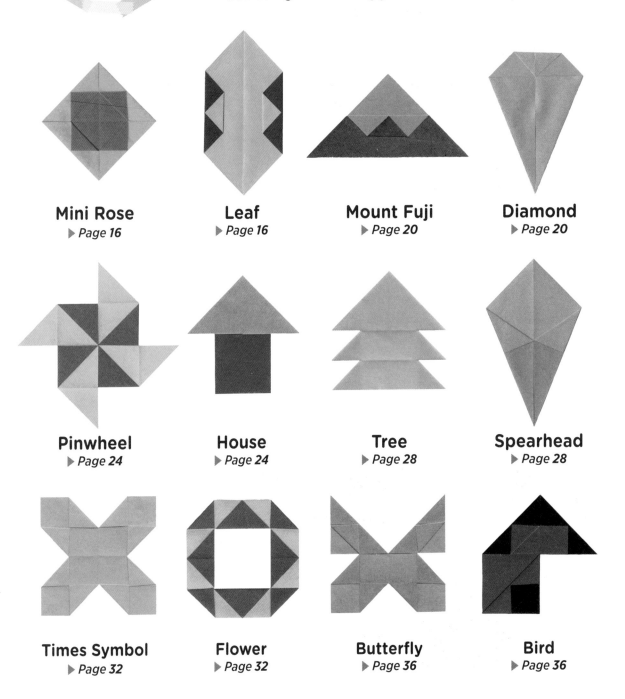

Mini Rose
▶ *Page 16*

Leaf
▶ *Page 16*

Mount Fuji
▶ *Page 20*

Diamond
▶ *Page 20*

Pinwheel
▶ *Page 24*

House
▶ *Page 24*

Tree
▶ *Page 28*

Spearhead
▶ *Page 28*

Times Symbol
▶ *Page 32*

Flower
▶ *Page 32*

Butterfly
▶ *Page 36*

Bird
▶ *Page 36*

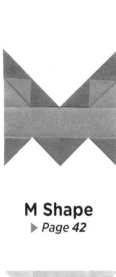

M Shape
▶ *Page 42*

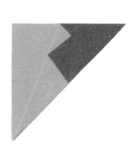

Boomerang
▶ *Page 42*

Arrowhead
▶ *Page 46*

Feather
▶ *Page 46*

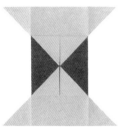

Drum
▶ *Page 50*

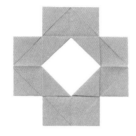

Plus Symbol
▶ *Page 50*

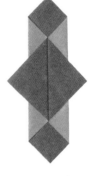

Necktie
▶ *Page 54*

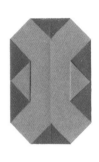

Oval Coin
▶ *Page 54*

Leaf Badge
▶ *Page 58*

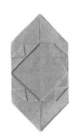

Gem
▶ *Page 58*

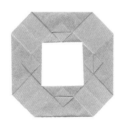

Prism
▶ *Page 62*

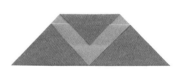

Trapezoid
▶ *Page 62*

Origami Butterfly
▶ *Page 69*

Tulip
▶ *Page 70*

Heart
▶ *Page 91*

Maple Leaf
▶ *Page 105*

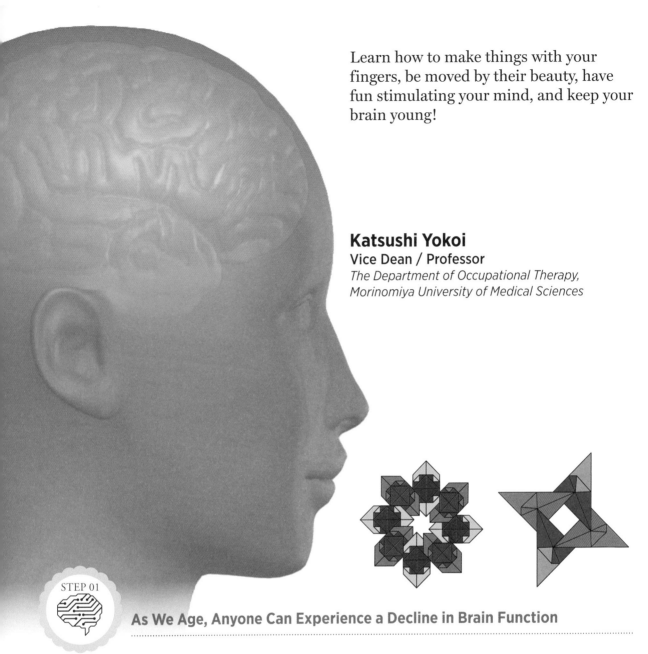

Learn how to make things with your fingers, be moved by their beauty, have fun stimulating your mind, and keep your brain young!

Katsushi Yokoi
Vice Dean / Professor
The Department of Occupational Therapy, Morinomiya University of Medical Sciences

STEP 01

As We Age, Anyone Can Experience a Decline in Brain Function

Having a brain that functions youthfully, where one's thoughts and words flow smoothly, is something everyone wishes to maintain throughout their lives. This capability is governed by what is called "cognitive function," which enables the brain to comprehend received information, process it, and respond accordingly.

Everyone tends to become more forgetful as the years roll by, but forgetting something and then remembering it with a hint should not be considered "dementia." Dementia is a progressive disease that occurs with aging, where various factors cause damage to brain cells, leading to impairments in cognitive functions and other areas. Memory loss caused by dementia involves events completely slipping away, making them impossible to recall even with hints.

Until a generation ago, dementia was considered unpreventable, but now, research is ongoing worldwide, and methods to decrease the odds of occurrence are becoming more well-understood.

The main preventative methods are:
1. Improving one's diet
2. Establishing exercise habits
3. Ensuring quality sleep
4. Training the brain

The origami presented in this book helps with the fourth method: brain training. Take a moment to evaluate your lifestyle in relation to the other prevention methods. In addition to these four methods, social contact is important because it builds the resilience known as "cognitive reserve."

STEP 02

Early Detection and Measures Against Cognitive Decline

Currently, the top three factors necessitating long-term care are: lifestyle-related cerebrovascular diseases, musculoskeletal disorders involving muscles, joints and bones, and dementia. The Japanese Ministry of Health, Labour and Welfare reported that, as of 2012, there were approximately 4.62 million people with dementia in Japan, meaning one in seven Japanese people over the age of 65 is affected. Furthermore, it is estimated that by 2025, when the Baby Boomer generation will be over 75 years old, one in five people over 65 will have dementia. This equates to a 1.5-fold increase over a span of only ten years or so.

While it is impossible to cure dementia with current medical technology, it is possible to slow its progression. Therefore, early detection and intervention are crucial. Mild Cognitive Impairment (MCI) is particularly noteworthy here. Recent research has revealed that before the onset of dementia, MCI is present.

Katsushi Yokoi

Professional Experience

1990 - Shitennoji Temple
1992 - Himeji St. Maria Hospital
1993 - Yumemae Rehabilitation Center
1994 - Medcare Rehabilitation Corporation
1997 - Kansai Medical Technology School
2001 - Kasei Medical Corporation
2009 - Himeji Dokkyo University
2013 - Kansai Welfare Science University
2016 - Research Fellow at Wakayama Medical University (present)

Publications

- *Community Rehabilitation Techniques* / Miwa Bookstore
- *Rehabilitation in Elderly Facilities* / Miwa Bookstore
- *Caregiver Training Series 2 "Life Support Techniques"* / Reiho Publishing
- *Exercises for Preventing Falls: Approaches to Motor and Cognitive Functions* / Miwa Bookstore
- *Introduction to Caregiving Practice: Caregiver Training Series Volume 5* / Reimei Bookstore

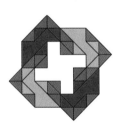 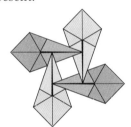 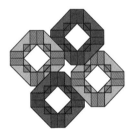 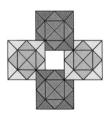

STEP 03

Dual-tasking Activates Various Parts of the Brain

Mild Cognitive Impairment represents a transition zone between healthy cognitive function and dementia, indicating a state where cognitive functions have declined more than is typical for one's age. If the condition is diagnosed while in the MCI stage, cognitive functions might improve with effective training.

Exercises known to enhance cognitive functions include aerobic activities such as walking, jogging and aqua walking. Adding brain training exercises, which are said to be highly effective in maintaining and improving cognitive skills, constitutes a "dual task."

Dual-tasking involves performing two tasks simultaneously. Engaging in conversation while walking represents one type of dual-tasking. In healthy individuals, dual-tasking is done effortlessly in daily life—for example, cooking while watching TV or folding laundry while singing. However, as cognitive function declines, one might accidentally burn their dinner while focusing on the TV, or drop out of a conversation while focusing on walking, or trip and fall while engrossed in a conversation. Many falls among the elderly are precipitated by cognitive decline, which makes it difficult to dual-task.

Let's consider an example of using dual-task training that is helpful for maintaining and improving cognitive function. In this instance, the training consists of:

Task 1: Walking in place
Task 2: Singing a newly learned song

The task of walking in place activates the part of the brain that controls body movement. Adding the task of singing a newly learned song stimulates memory and attention. Performing such dual tasks is said to activate various parts of the brain and enhance cognitive abilities.

STEP 04

Make it Your Practice to Create Beautiful Crafts to Keep Your Brain Vibrant

Folding modular origami is considered an effective form of dual-task training. You look at diagrams, read and understand the text, choose paper colors, fold with your fingertips, assemble, and decorate. In addition, by showing it to others and talking about it, social connections are strengthened.

By making it a habit to create beautiful crafts, the kind of stimulation that preserves the youthfulness of one's brain also becomes ingrained. It's fun to do, and therefore it's easy to repeat, and continuing to do it makes it effective. Keep at it, and trust in the power of persistence!

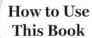

How to Use This Book

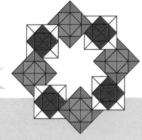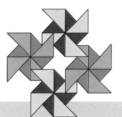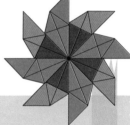

● **Aim for about 20 minutes of crafting time every day.**

Overexerting yourself to the point of fatigue is counterproductive for the brain. Try to enjoy it as a daily routine at roughly the same time each day, which will help to establish it as a habit. It's okay if you don't finish the artwork and leave it incomplete; you can just continue with it the next time.

● **After you create the individual parts, assembling them into a finished product is presented as a "challenge."**

Don't immediately look up the methods that solve the challenges. Instead, we encourage you to observe, innovate, and engage in trial and error so you can enjoy finding the solutions on your own.

The different methods of combining the parts enable you to create many configurations beyond those introduced here. Try out all sorts of ideas!

● **Discuss the enjoyable aspects of folding origami, what kinds of artwork you created, and how you thought about the decorations with your family and friends.**

Origami can be a wonderful conversation starter, providing opportunities to chat and expanding your social circle.

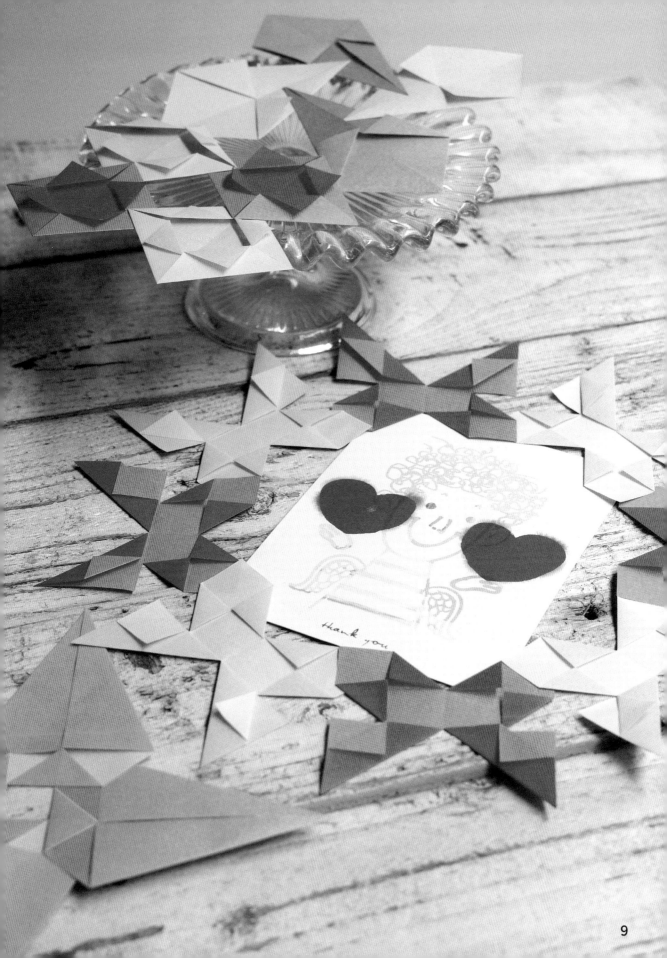

thank you

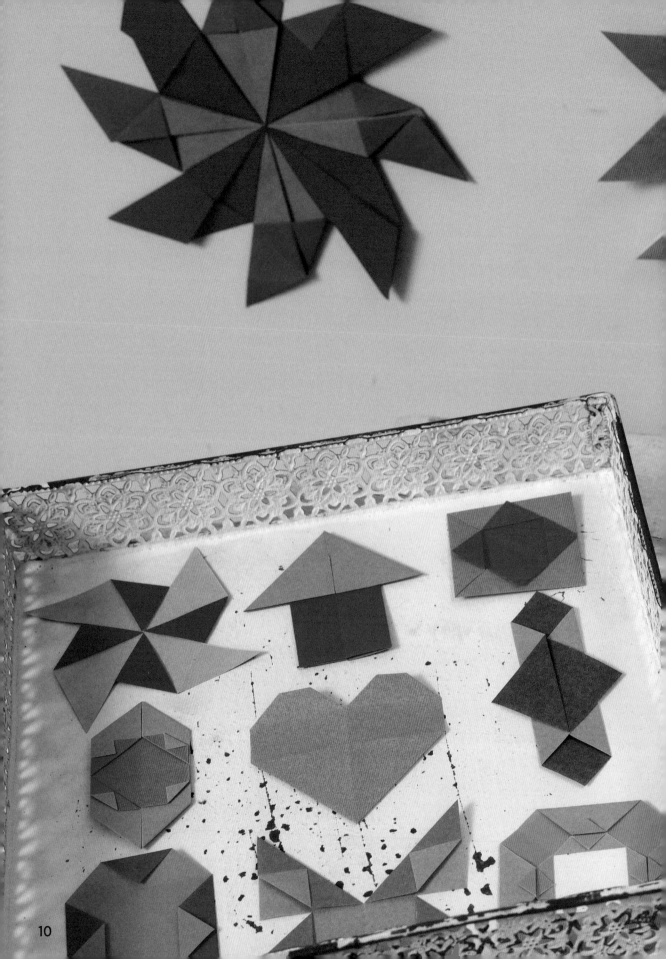

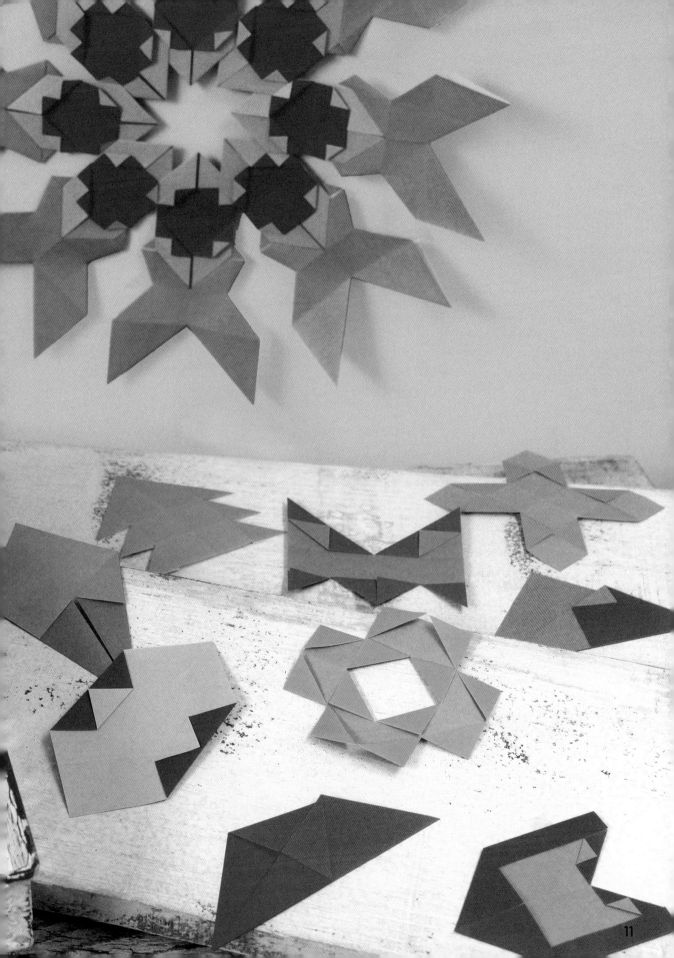

When creating papercrafts, it's essential to know how to choose your paper, use the tools, and understand the folding methods and combination techniques. These basic concepts may be simple, but they are crucial keys to completing your projects in a beautiful and satisfactory way. Please take a few moments to learn them.

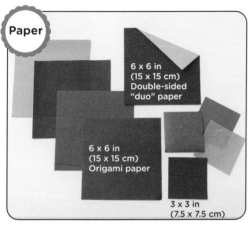

Paper

6 x 6 in (15 x 15 cm) Double-sided "duo" paper

6 x 6 in (15 x 15 cm) Origami paper

3 x 3 in (7.5 x 7.5 cm)

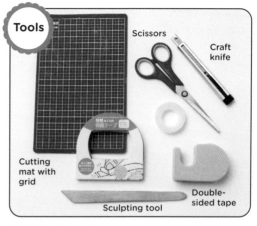

Tools

Scissors

Craft knife

Cutting mat with grid

Double-sided tape

Sculpting tool

We start with 6 inch (15 cm) squares of commercially available origami papers. Unless specifically directed to use a different paper size, prepare your paper by folding one of these sheets into quarters, and then cutting along the creases to yield four 3 inch (7.5 cm) squares, which will be the standard size used for folding the parts. You can also purchase origami paper already cut to the 3 inch (7.5 cm) size.

One type of origami paper has only one side that is colored, and then there is "double-sided" (or "duo") paper, which has a different color on each side. Choose paper according to the theme of your work, or your preference.

Grid-lined Work Mat
Working on a grid-lined mat helps you assemble parts neatly, as it enables you to align them horizontally or vertically. It's also very useful for measuring consistent lengths and angles.

Double-sided Tape/Transparent Tape
Using liquid or stick glue to adhere parts can cause the paper to absorb moisture and wrinkle. To avoid this, all assembly in this book is done with double-sided or transparent tape.

Sculpting Tool (like those used for clay modeling, available at stationery stores):
After folding the paper, tracing and pressing down the crease with a sculpting tool ensures a sharp fold. This tool is essential to keep the shape of your artwork stable.

Scissors/Cutter
Choose whatever is comfortable for you. A cutter is handy for cutting paper, especially if you have a ruler.

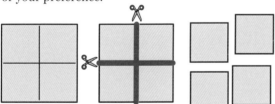

Paper Folding Methods

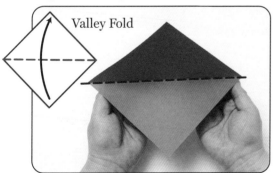

Valley Fold

Pull the edges toward you to fold, finishing with the valley crease on the inside.

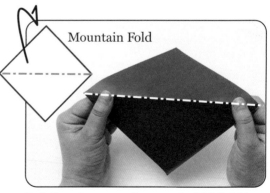

Mountain Fold

Push the edges away from you to fold, finishing with the mountain crease on the outside.

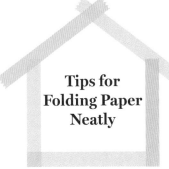

Tips for Folding Paper Neatly

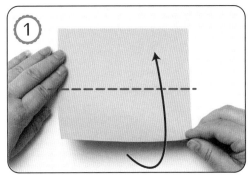

Hold one edge of the paper and, instead of creasing immediately, bend the entire sheet gently in half.

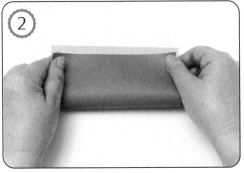

Carefully align the edges.

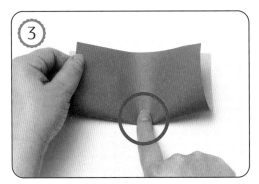

Press down in the center with your finger.

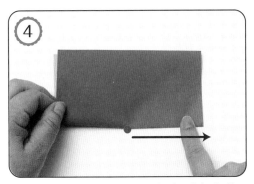

Slide your finger to crease only the right half.

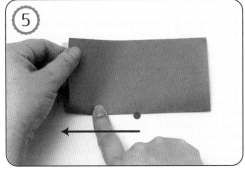

Press the center again and slide your finger to crease the left half.

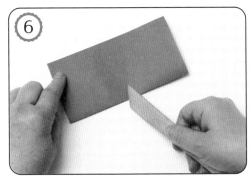

Use a wooden sculpting tool to trace and sharpen the crease.

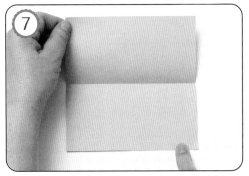

This results in a crisp, sharp fold.

How to Attach the Parts to Construct Compositions

....

The Basics of Modular Origami

When attaching overlapping parts together, use double-sided tape. When connecting the edges of parts, use transparent tape. In this book, the focus is on compositions consisting of 4 or 8 parts in a circular arrangement. An important aspect the final steps is to swap the first part used with the last part attached so that the first part ends up on top.

Affixing Parts with Double-sided Tape

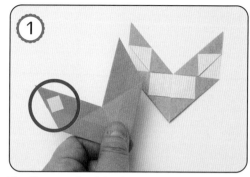

The first part is pink. Place a square of double-sided tape on the back side of the overlapping area of the second part, which is blue.

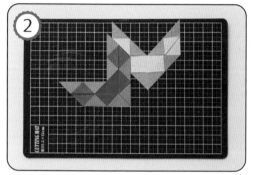

On a grid-lined work mat, align the parts horizontally and vertically as you attach them together.

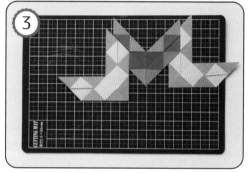

Continue attaching parts in the same way, gradually forming a circle.

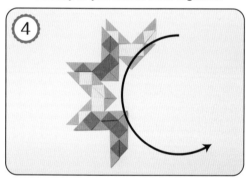

Stack and attach the parts in a counterclockwise direction.

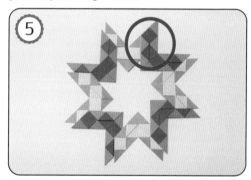

Now, prepare to complete the circle. In this photo, the first part is under the last part.

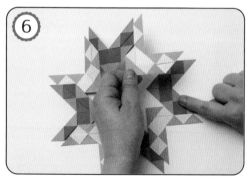

Pull the first part out from under the last part and place it on top.

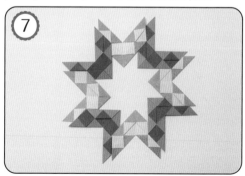

Attach double-sided tape to the back of the first part, connect it to the last part to complete the circle, and the piece is completed.

Affixing Parts with Transparent Tape

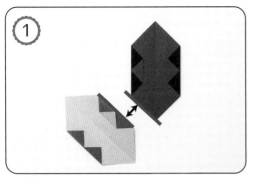

The first part is red-black. Connect it edge to edge with the second part, which is yellow-brown.

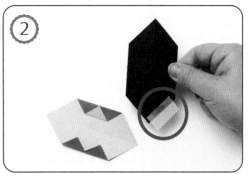

Apply a strip of transparent tape to the back of the red-black part, spanning the edge that will be connected.

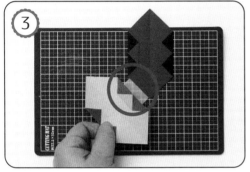

On a grid-lined work mat, align the parts horizontally and vertically as you attach them together.

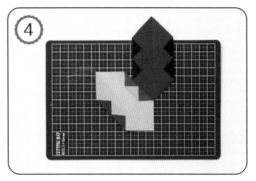

Place the second part on top of the transparent tape to adhere it. Aligning it with the grid ensures there is no misalignment.

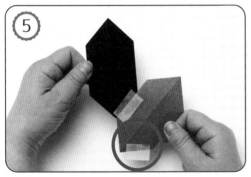

Apply transparent tape on the back.

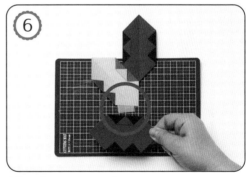

Align the parts together.

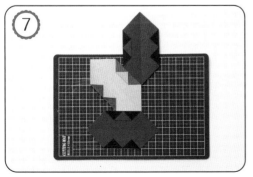

Continue attaching and adding parts in the same manner, gradually forming a circle.

Mini Rose

This square part can look like a small rose or the calyx of a flower. A key to finishing it beautifully is to precisely align the four corners at the center of the paper when folding.

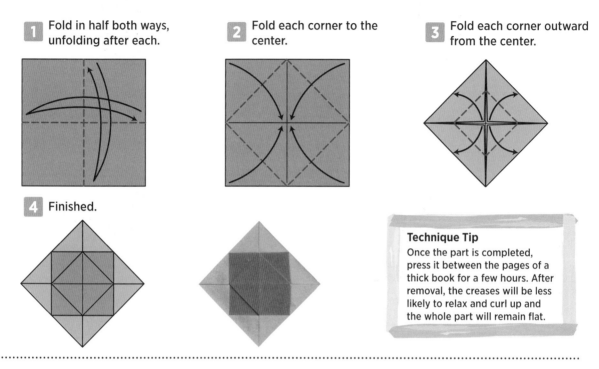

1 Fold in half both ways, unfolding after each.

2 Fold each corner to the center.

3 Fold each corner outward from the center.

4 Finished.

Technique Tip
Once the part is completed, press it between the pages of a thick book for a few hours. After removal, the creases will be less likely to relax and curl up and the whole part will remain flat.

Leaf

Depending on your choice of paper color, this part can resemble fresh green leaves or be suitable for a holiday poinsettia. Practice to perfect aligning the corners at the center of the paper in step 2.

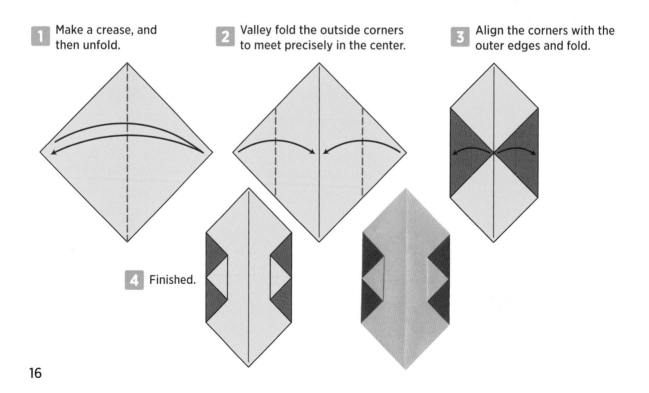

1 Make a crease, and then unfold.

2 Valley fold the outside corners to meet precisely in the center.

3 Align the corners with the outer edges and fold.

4 Finished.

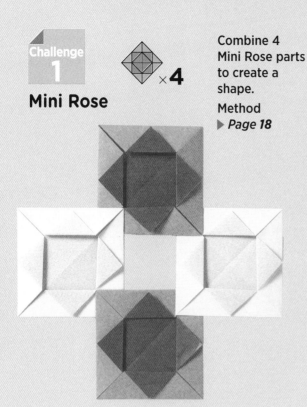

×4

Combine 4 Mini Rose parts to create a shape.
Method
▶ *Page 18*

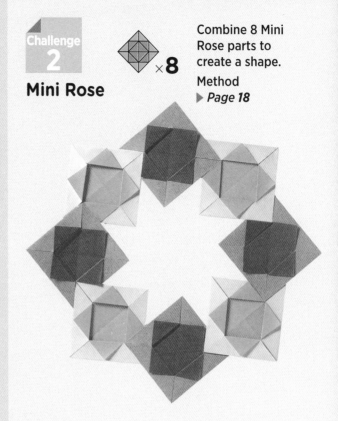

×8

Combine 8 Mini Rose parts to create a shape.
Method
▶ *Page 18*

While chatting with friends, fold up parts and join them together, and "flowers" will soon bloom on the wall!

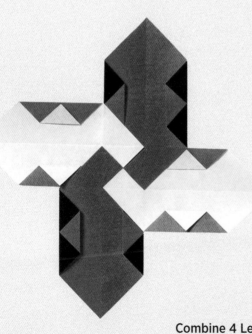

Combine 4 Leaf parts to create a shape.
Method
▶ *Page 19*

Challenge
3

Leaf

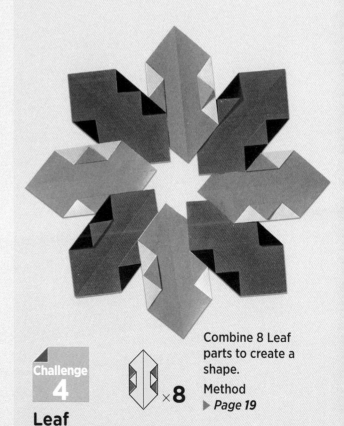

×4

Combine 8 Leaf parts to create a shape.
Method
▶ *Page 19*

Challenge
4

Leaf

×8

17

Methods for
Mini Rose Challenges

 ×**4**

 ×**8**

Challenge ▶ *Page 17*

Challenge ▶ *Page 17*

1 Superimpose the second part on the lower left corner of the first part, aligning it to the blue dashed line. Adhere the parts together.

1 Superimpose the second part on the lower left area of the first part, aligning it to the blue dashed line. Adhere the parts together.

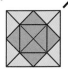

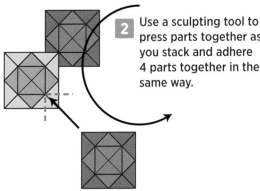

2 Use a sculpting tool to press parts together as you stack and adhere 4 parts together in the same way.

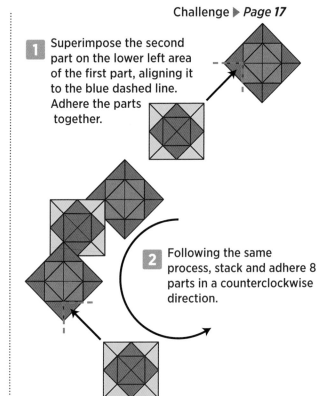

2 Following the same process, stack and adhere 8 parts in a counterclockwise direction.

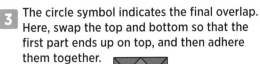

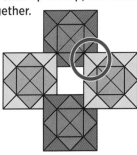

3 The circle symbol indicates the final overlap. Here, swap the top and bottom so that the first part ends up on top, and then adhere them together.

3 The circle symbol indicates the final overlap. Here, swap the top and bottom so that the first part ends up on top, and then adhere them together.

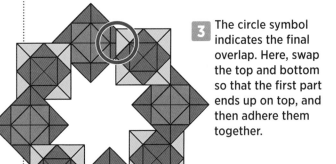

4 Finished.

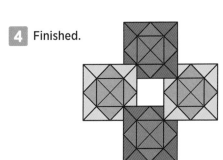

4 Finished.

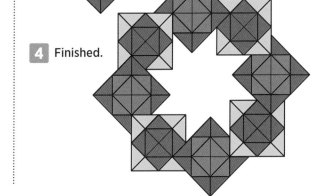

18

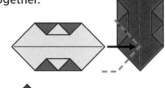 ×**4**

Methods for
Leaf Challenges

  ×**8**

Challenge ▶ *Page 17*

Challenge ▶ *Page 17*

1 Superimpose the second part on the lower left area of the first part, aligning it to the blue dashed line. Adhere the parts together.

1 Superimpose the second part on the lower left area of the first part, aligning it to the blue dashed line. Adhere the parts together.

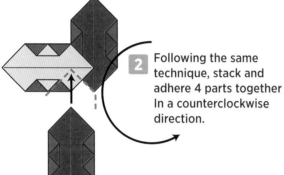

2 Following the same technique, stack and adhere 4 parts together In a counterclockwise direction.

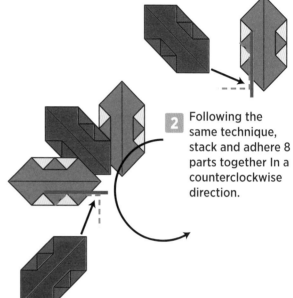

2 Following the same technique, stack and adhere 8 parts together In a counterclockwise direction.

3 The oval symbol indicates the final overlap. Here, swap the top and bottom so that the first part ends up on top, and then adhere them together.

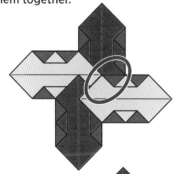

3 The oval symbol indicates the final overlap. Here, swap the top and bottom so that the first part ends up on top, and then adhere them together.

4 Finished.

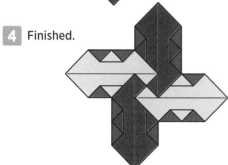

4 Finished.

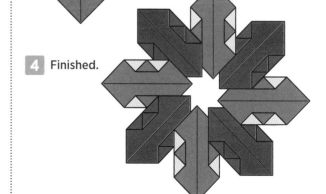

Mount Fuji

The key to a neat finish is to precisely fold down the top layer so that the corner touches the bottom edge, as shown in step 3. Although there are no landmarks, you need to bring the corner to a position that evenly divides the length of the bottom edge into left and right sections.

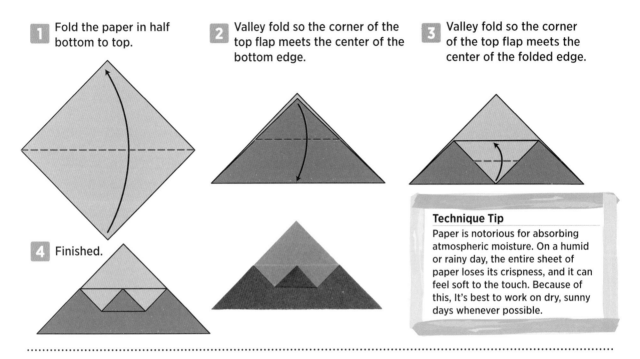

1 Fold the paper in half bottom to top.

2 Valley fold so the corner of the top flap meets the center of the bottom edge.

3 Valley fold so the corner of the top flap meets the center of the folded edge.

4 Finished.

Technique Tip
Paper is notorious for absorbing atmospheric moisture. On a humid or rainy day, the entire sheet of paper loses its crispness, and it can feel soft to the touch. Because of this, It's best to work on dry, sunny days whenever possible.

Diamond

When you align the lower edges to the central vertical crease in step 2, be sure that the newly formed horizontal edges meet to form a straight line, as indicated by the purple line shown at step 3.

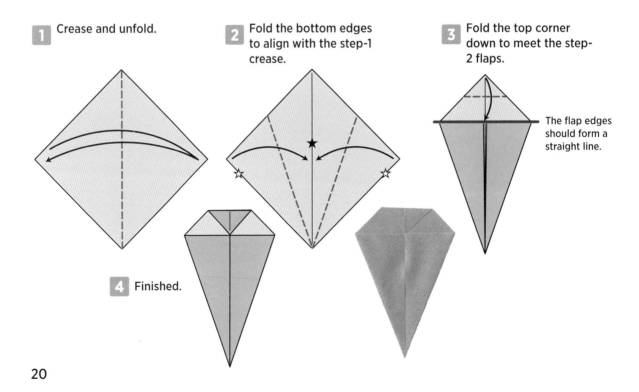

1 Crease and unfold.

2 Fold the bottom edges to align with the step-1 crease.

3 Fold the top corner down to meet the step-2 flaps.

The flap edges should form a straight line.

4 Finished.

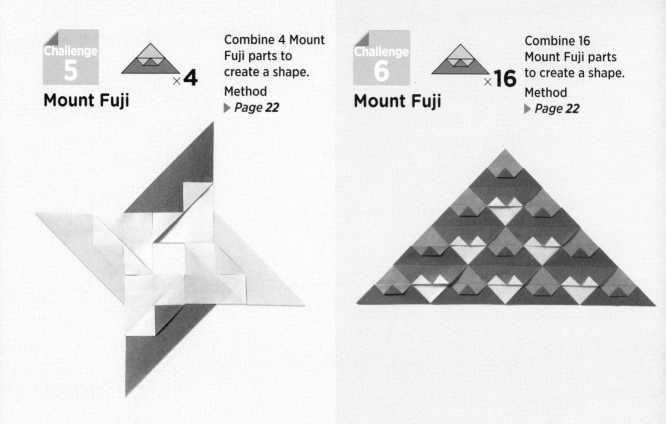

Challenge 5

Mount Fuji

×4

Combine 4 Mount Fuji parts to create a shape.
Method
▶ *Page 22*

Challenge 6

Mount Fuji

×16

Combine 16 Mount Fuji parts to create a shape.
Method
▶ *Page 22*

The look of the finished piece changes significantly depending on the paper you've selected. Try making and comparing assemblages with different colors.

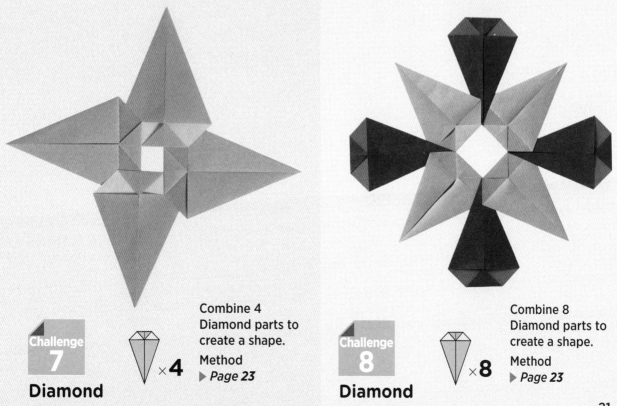

Challenge 7

Diamond

×4

Combine 4 Diamond parts to create a shape.
Method
▶ *Page 23*

Challenge 8

Diamond

×8

Combine 8 Diamond parts to create a shape.
Method
▶ *Page 23*

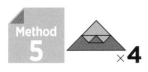

Method 5 ×**4**

Challenge ▶ *Page 21*

1 Superimpose the second part on the lower left corner of the first part, aligning it to the blue dashed line. Adhere the parts together.

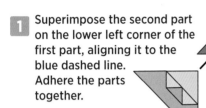

2 Repeat for 4 parts in total, arranging and adhering them together as shown.

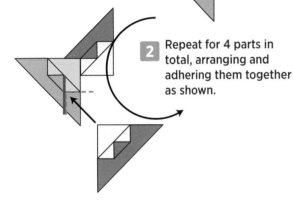

3 The circle symbol indicates the final overlap. Here, swap the top and bottom so that the first part ends up on top, and then adhere them together.

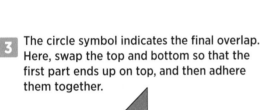

4 Finished.

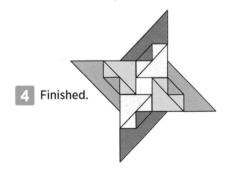

Method 6 ×**16**

Challenge ▶ *Page 21*

1 Align the bases of 2 triangles, and tape them together on the back. Make 6 identical sets.

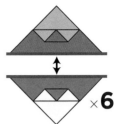

×**6**

2 Combine the 6 sets, align the edges, and tape them together to form a pyramid shape.

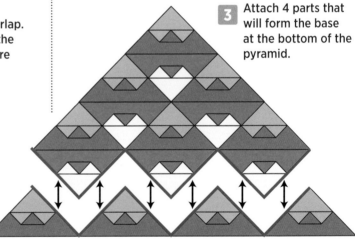

3 Attach 4 parts that will form the base at the bottom of the pyramid.

4 Finished.

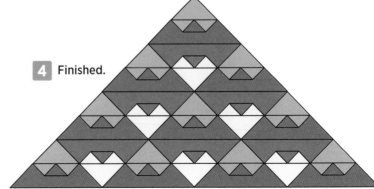

Method 7 ×**4**

Methods for
Diamond Challenges

Method 8 ×**8**

Challenge ▸ *Page 21*

1 Superimpose the second part on the lower left area of the first part, aligning it to the blue dashed line. Adhere the parts together.

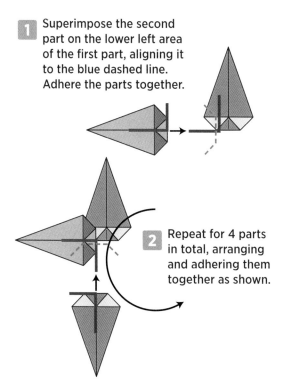

2 Repeat for 4 parts in total, arranging and adhering them together as shown.

3 The circle symbol indicates the final overlap. Here, swap the top and bottom so that the first part ends up on top, and then adhere them together.

4 Finished.

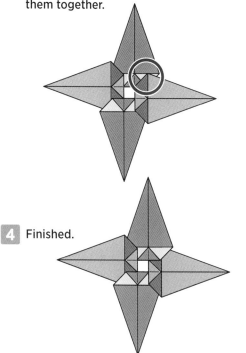

Challenge ▸ *Page 21*

1 Rotate the second part as shown, then superimpose the second part on the lower left area of the first part, aligning it to the blue dashed line. Adhere the parts together.

2 Rotate the second part as shown. Align as shown, and adhere the parts together.

3 Repeat with 8 parts in total, arranging and adhering them together as shown.

4 The circle symbol indicates the final overlap. Here, swap the top and bottom so that the first part ends up on top, and then adhere together.

5 Finished.

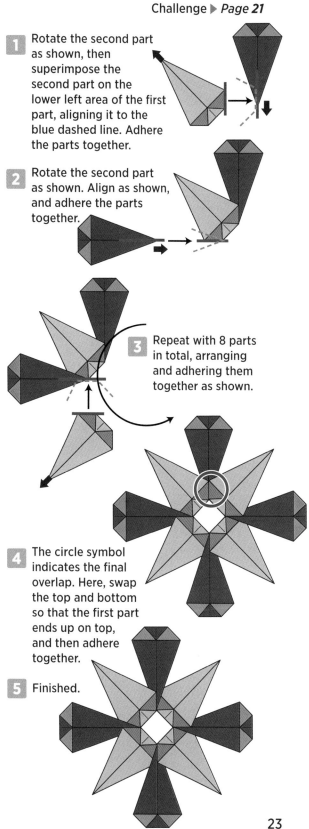

Pinwheel

While you'll make many creases here, only 4 triangular flaps remain folded to create the shape. Attaching double-sided tape to the back of these four triangular flaps will prevent the paper from lifting, making it easier to handle.

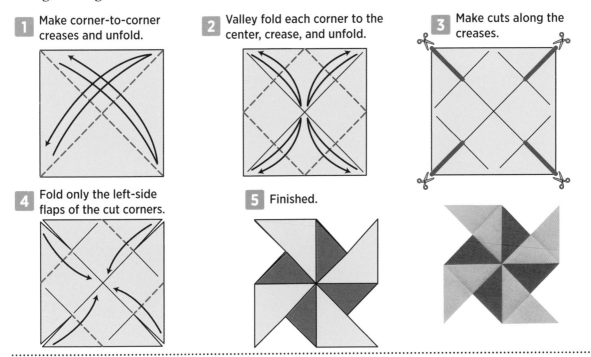

1 Make corner-to-corner creases and unfold.

2 Valley fold each corner to the center, crease, and unfold.

3 Make cuts along the creases.

4 Fold only the left-side flaps of the cut corners.

5 Finished.

House

The colors on the front and back of the paper will be split between the roof and the lower part in the finished piece. The choice of paper colors will determine the look of the assembled Challenge compositions. Carefully consider the color schemes based on your preferences.

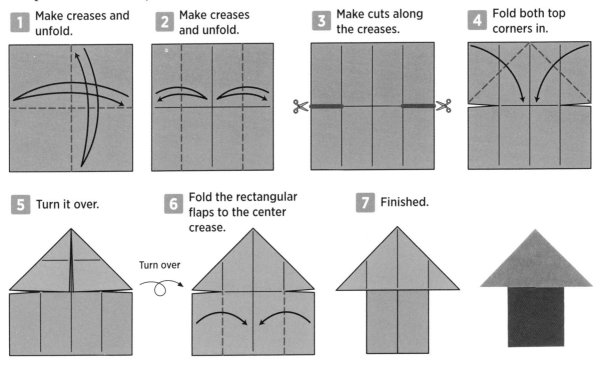

1 Make creases and unfold.

2 Make creases and unfold.

3 Make cuts along the creases.

4 Fold both top corners in.

5 Turn it over.

Turn over

6 Fold the rectangular flaps to the center crease.

7 Finished.

Challenge 9

Pinwheel

 ×4

Combine 4 Pinwheel parts to create a shape.

Method
▶ *Page 26*

Challenge 10

Pinwheel

 ×8

Combine 8 Pinwheel parts to create a shape.

Method
▶ *Page 26*

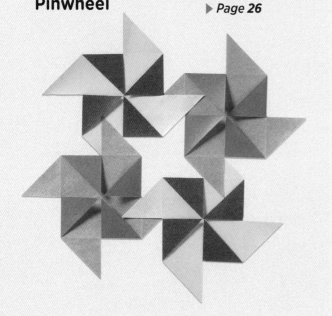

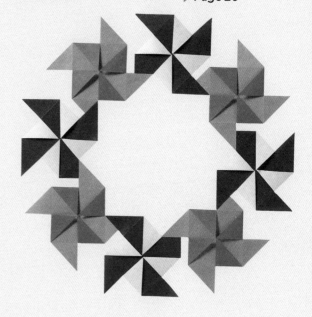

These pieces appear ready to spin in the wind.
When assembled, they express a pleasing harmony.

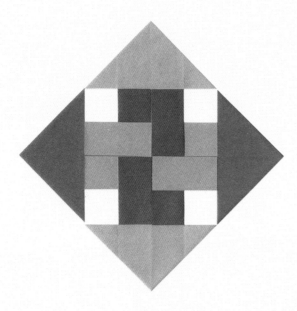

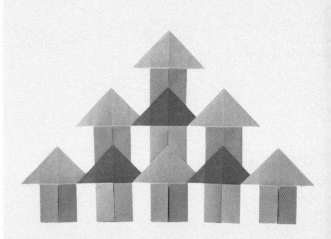

Challenge 11

 ×4

House

Combine 4 House parts to create a shape.

Method
▶ *Page 27*

Challenge 12

 ×9

House

Combine 9 House parts to create a shape.

Method
▶ *Page 27*

Methods for
Pinwheel Challenges

Challenge ▶ *Page 25*

Challenge ▶ *Page 25*

1 Superimpose the second part on the first part, aligning it to the blue dashed line. Adhere the parts together.

1 Superimpose the second part on the lower left corner of the first part, aligning it to the blue dashed line. Adhere the parts together.

2 Repeat for 4 parts in total, arranging and adhering them together as shown.

2 Repeat for 8 parts in total, arranging and adhering them together as shown.

3 The circle symbol indicates the final overlap. Here, swap the top and bottom so that the first part ends up on top, and then adhere together.

3 The circle symbol indicates the final overlap. Here, swap the top and bottom so that the first part ends up on top, and then adhere them together.

4 Finished.

4 Finished.

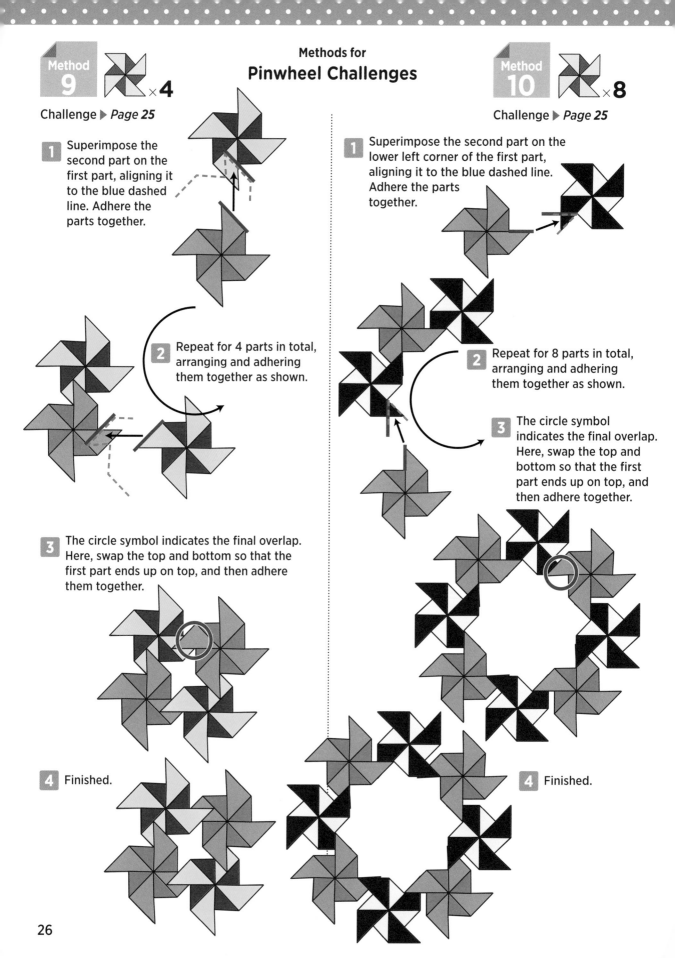

26

House Challenges

Method 11 ×4

Challenge ▶ *Page 25*

1 Superimpose the second part on the lower left corner of the first part, aligning it to the blue dashed line. Adhere the parts together.

2 Repeat for 4 parts in total, arranging and adhering them together as shown.

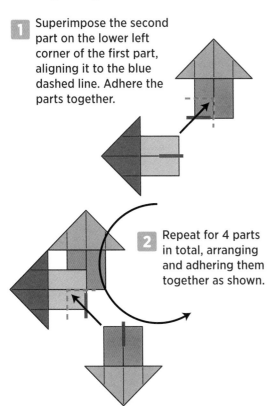

3 The circle symbol indicates the final overlap. Here, swap the top and bottom so that the first part ends up on top, and then adhere them together.

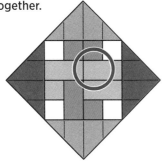

4 Finished.

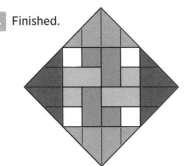

Method 12 ×9

Challenge ▶ *Page 25*

1 Place the second part under the bottom of the first part, aligning it to the blue dashed line. Adhere the parts together.

2 Arrange 3 parts horizontally, with the circle-symbol corners on top, and adhere them together.

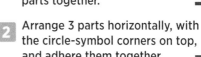
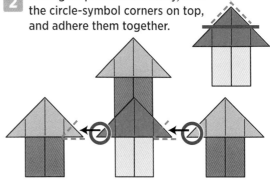

3 In the same manner, arrange 5 parts horizontally, and adhere them together.

Superimpose the 5-part assembly, and adhere the sections together to form a pyramid shape.

4 Finished.

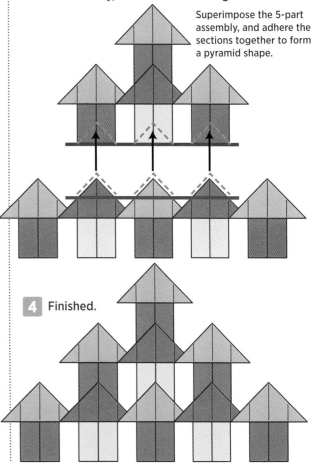

Tree

The finished product will only show the color on one side (the front) of the paper. Therefore, you do not need to use double-sided origami paper with colors on both sides for this part.

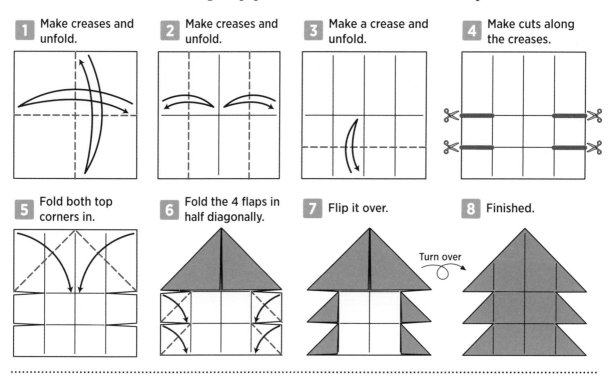

1 Make creases and unfold.

2 Make creases and unfold.

3 Make a crease and unfold.

4 Make cuts along the creases.

5 Fold both top corners in.

6 Fold the 4 flaps in half diagonally.

7 Flip it over.

Turn over

8 Finished.

Spearhead

This part looks like the business end of a spear, but in the origami composition on page 72, it is used as a bouquet wrapper. What you imagine from its shape is up to you.

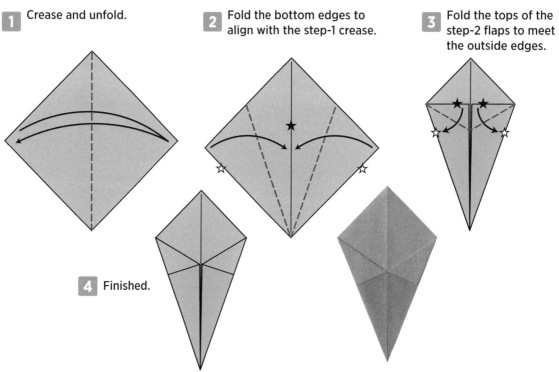

1 Crease and unfold.

2 Fold the bottom edges to align with the step-1 crease.

3 Fold the tops of the step-2 flaps to meet the outside edges.

4 Finished.

Challenge 13

Tree

×4

Combine 4 Tree parts to create a shape.
Method
▶ *Page 30*

Challenge 14

Tree

×6

Combine 6 Tree parts to create a shape.
Method
▶ *Page 30*

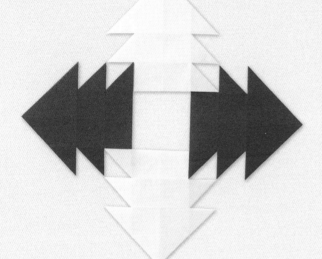

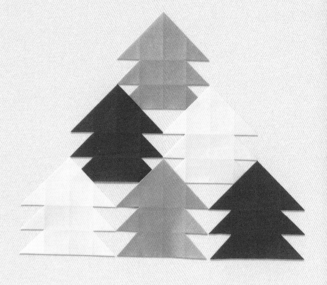

As you make multiple parts,
you will begin to establish "muscle memory."

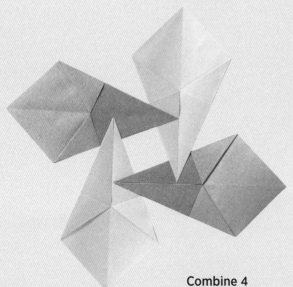

Combine 4 Spearhead parts to create a shape.
Method
▶ *Page 31*

Challenge 15

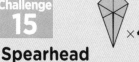×4

Spearhead

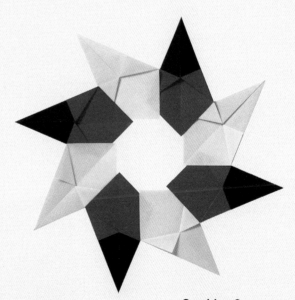

Combine 8 Spearhead parts to create a shape.
Method
▶ *Page 31*

Challenge 16

×8

Spearhead

Methods for
Tree Challenges

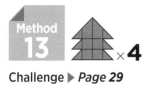×**4**

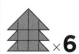×**6**

Challenge ▶ *Page 29*

Challenge ▶ *Page 29*

1 Superimpose the second part on the lower left corner of the first part, aligning it to the blue dashed line. Adhere the parts together.

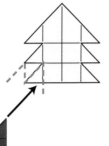

2 Repeat for 4 parts in total, arranging and adhering them together as shown.

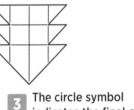
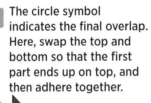

3 The circle symbol indicates the final overlap. Here, swap the top and bottom so that the first part ends up on top, and then adhere together.

4 Finished.

1 Superimpose 2 parts on the bottom corners of the first part, align them as shown and adhere them together.

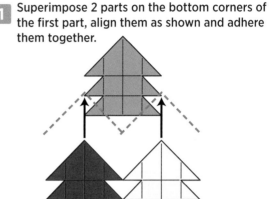

2 Superimpose 3 parts over the step-1 assembly to form a pyramid shape. Align as indicated and adhere the parts together.

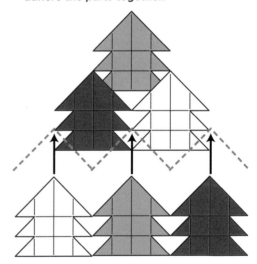

3 Finished.

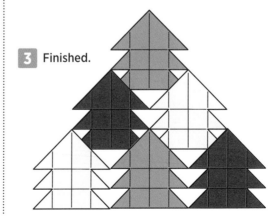

Methods for
Spearhead Challenges

Method 15 ×4

Challenge ▶ *Page 29*

Method 16 ×8

Challenge ▶ *Page 29*

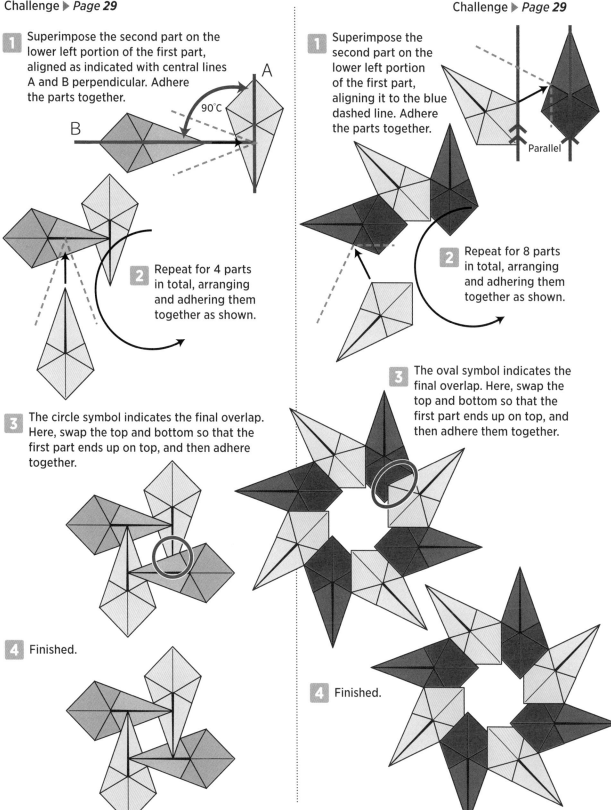

1 Superimpose the second part on the lower left portion of the first part, aligned as indicated with central lines A and B perpendicular. Adhere the parts together.

90°C

A

B

2 Repeat for 4 parts in total, arranging and adhering them together as shown.

3 The circle symbol indicates the final overlap. Here, swap the top and bottom so that the first part ends up on top, and then adhere together.

4 Finished.

1 Superimpose the second part on the lower left portion of the first part, aligning it to the blue dashed line. Adhere the parts together.

Parallel

2 Repeat for 8 parts in total, arranging and adhering them together as shown.

3 The oval symbol indicates the final overlap. Here, swap the top and bottom so that the first part ends up on top, and then adhere them together.

4 Finished.

31

Times Symbol

This shape enables you to enjoy various ways of connecting the parts. In the "challenges," they are arranged in circles, but you can also align them vertically or stack them into a pyramid shape for a beautiful result.

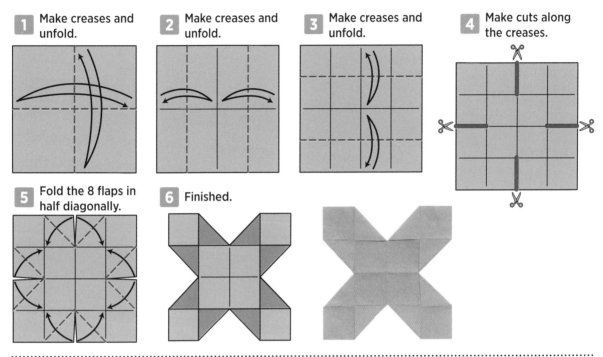

1 Make creases and unfold.

2 Make creases and unfold.

3 Make creases and unfold.

4 Make cuts along the creases.

5 Fold the 8 flaps in half diagonally.

6 Finished.

Flower

Although the geometry of this shape is comprised of straight lines, when viewed together, they appear to form a circle, similar to the petals of a flower. The human mind is fascinating.

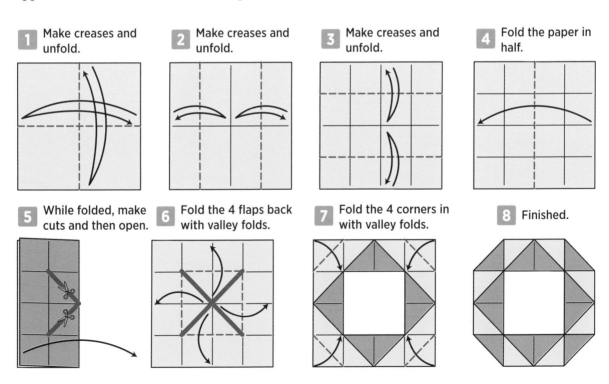

1 Make creases and unfold.

2 Make creases and unfold.

3 Make creases and unfold.

4 Fold the paper in half.

5 While folded, make cuts and then open.

6 Fold the 4 flaps back with valley folds.

7 Fold the 4 corners in with valley folds.

8 Finished.

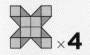

Combine 4 Times Symbol parts to create a shape.
Method
▶ *Page 34*

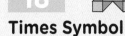
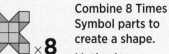

Combine 8 Times Symbol parts to create a shape.
Method
▶ *Page 34*

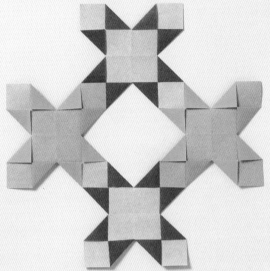

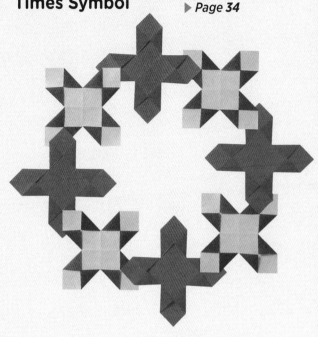

Pay attention to the shape of the "window" created by the surrounding parts.
A fascinating shape forms as you assemble the pieces.

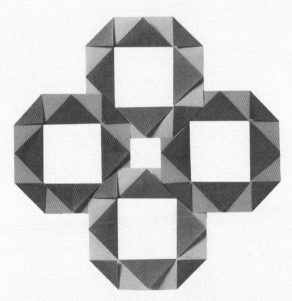

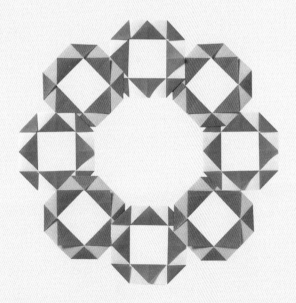

Challenge 19

Flower

Combine 4 Flower parts to create a shape.
Method
▶ *Page 35*

Challenge 20

Flower

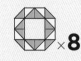

Combine 8 Flower parts to create a shape.
Method
▶ *Page 35*

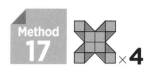

Method 17 ×**4**

Challenge ▶ *Page 33*

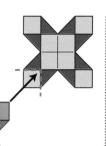

1 Superimpose the second part on the lower left corner of the first part, aligning it to the blue dashed line. Adhere the parts together.

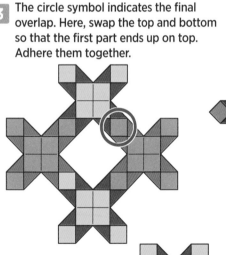

2 Repeat for 4 parts in total, arranging and adhering them together as shown.

3 The circle symbol indicates the final overlap. Here, swap the top and bottom so that the first part ends up on top. Adhere them together.

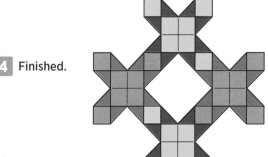

4 Finished.

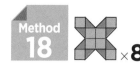

Method 18 ×**8**

Challenge ▶ *Page 33*

1 Superimpose the second part on the first part, aligning it as indicated. Adhere the parts together.

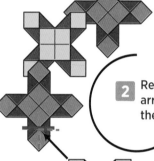

2 Repeat for 8 parts in total, arranging and adhering them together as shown.

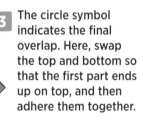

3 The circle symbol indicates the final overlap. Here, swap the top and bottom so that the first part ends up on top, and then adhere them together.

4 Finished.

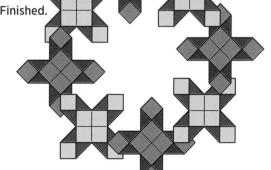

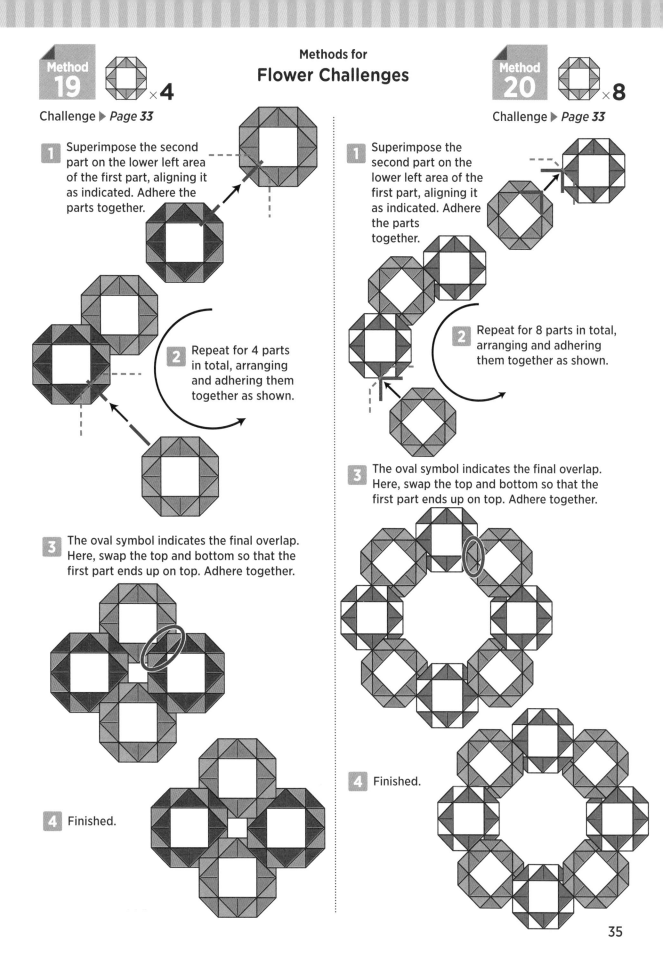

Methods for Flower Challenges

Method 19 ×4

Challenge ▶ *Page 33*

1 Superimpose the second part on the lower left area of the first part, aligning it as indicated. Adhere the parts together.

2 Repeat for 4 parts in total, arranging and adhering them together as shown.

3 The oval symbol indicates the final overlap. Here, swap the top and bottom so that the first part ends up on top. Adhere together.

4 Finished.

Method 20 ×8

Challenge ▶ *Page 33*

1 Superimpose the second part on the lower left area of the first part, aligning it as indicated. Adhere the parts together.

2 Repeat for 8 parts in total, arranging and adhering them together as shown.

3 The oval symbol indicates the final overlap. Here, swap the top and bottom so that the first part ends up on top. Adhere together.

4 Finished.

Butterfly

Through some clever folding, you can create a butterfly adorned with geometric patterns. When making cuts, use the base of the scissor blades rather than the tips for uninterrupted straight lines.

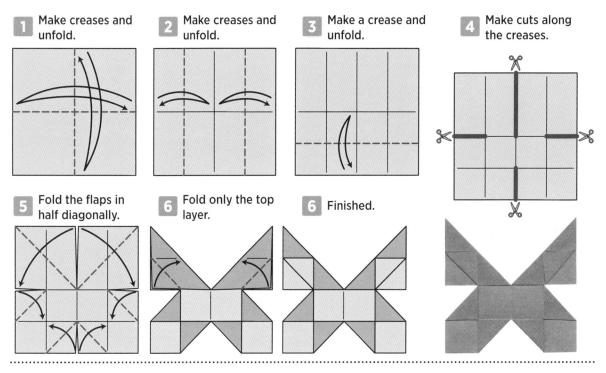

1 Make creases and unfold.

2 Make creases and unfold.

3 Make a crease and unfold.

4 Make cuts along the creases.

5 Fold the flaps in half diagonally.

6 Fold only the top layer.

6 Finished.

Bird

By combining several of these parts, mysterious and beautiful kaleidoscopic patterns emerge. The "windows" created by the parts form unexpected shapes.

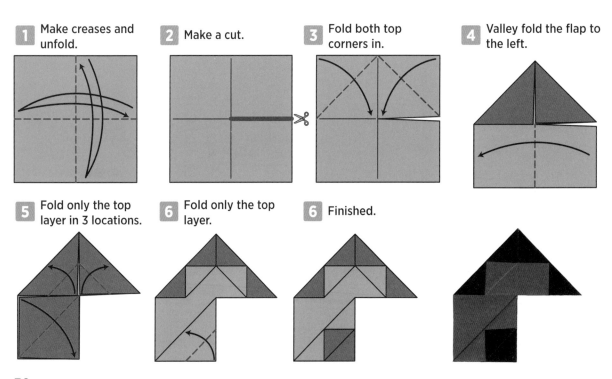

1 Make creases and unfold.

2 Make a cut.

3 Fold both top corners in.

4 Valley fold the flap to the left.

5 Fold only the top layer in 3 locations.

6 Fold only the top layer.

6 Finished.

Challenge 21

Butterfly

Combine 4 Butterfly parts to create a shape.
Method
▶ *Page 38*

 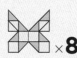

Challenge 22

Butterfly

Combine 8 Butterfly parts to create a shape.
Method
▶ *Page 38*

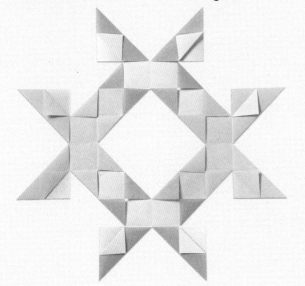

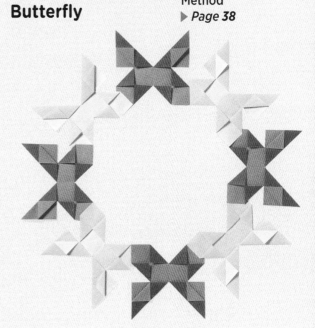

Use colorful origami frames to decorate photos or postcards inside the shapes.

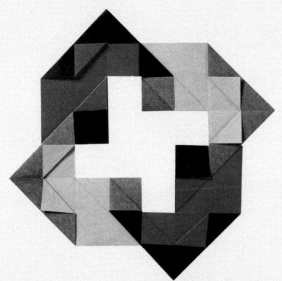

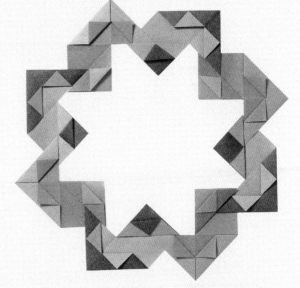

Challenge 23

Bird

Combine 4 Bird parts to create a shape.
Method
▶ *Page 39*

Challenge 24

Bird

Combine 8 Bird parts to create a shape.
Method
▶ *Page 39*

Methods for
Butterfly Challenges

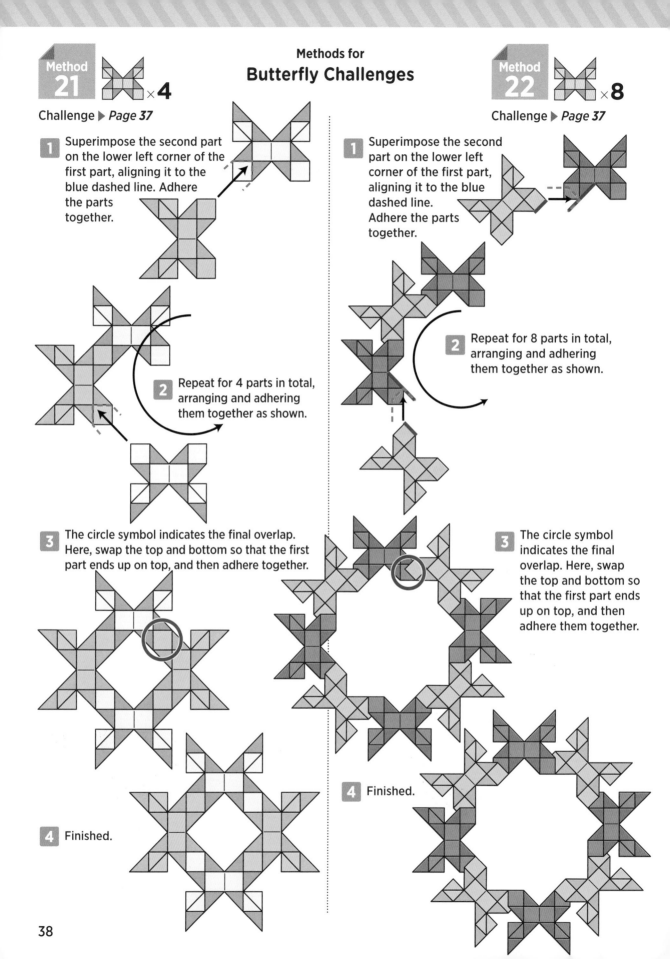

Method 21 ×4

Challenge ▶ *Page 37*

1 Superimpose the second part on the lower left corner of the first part, aligning it to the blue dashed line. Adhere the parts together.

2 Repeat for 4 parts in total, arranging and adhering them together as shown.

3 The circle symbol indicates the final overlap. Here, swap the top and bottom so that the first part ends up on top, and then adhere together.

4 Finished.

Method 22 ×8

Challenge ▶ *Page 37*

1 Superimpose the second part on the lower left corner of the first part, aligning it to the blue dashed line. Adhere the parts together.

2 Repeat for 8 parts in total, arranging and adhering them together as shown.

3 The circle symbol indicates the final overlap. Here, swap the top and bottom so that the first part ends up on top, and then adhere them together.

4 Finished.

Methods for
Bird Challenges

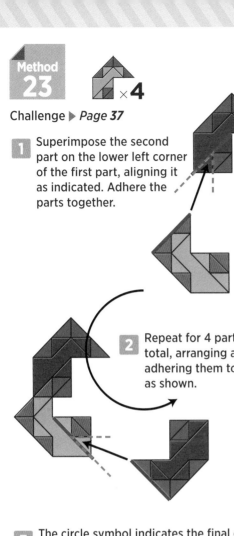

Method 23 ×4

Challenge ▶ *Page 37*

1 Superimpose the second part on the lower left corner of the first part, aligning it as indicated. Adhere the parts together.

2 Repeat for 4 parts in total, arranging and adhering them together as shown.

3 The circle symbol indicates the final overlap. Here, swap the top and bottom so that the first part ends up on top, and then adhere them together.

4 Finished.

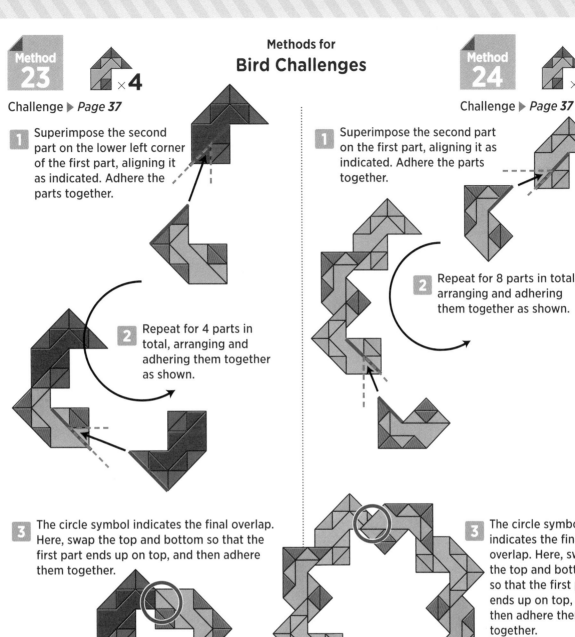

Method 24 ×8

Challenge ▶ *Page 37*

1 Superimpose the second part on the first part, aligning it as indicated. Adhere the parts together.

2 Repeat for 8 parts in total, arranging and adhering them together as shown.

3 The circle symbol indicates the final overlap. Here, swap the top and bottom so that the first part ends up on top, and then adhere them together.

4 Finished.

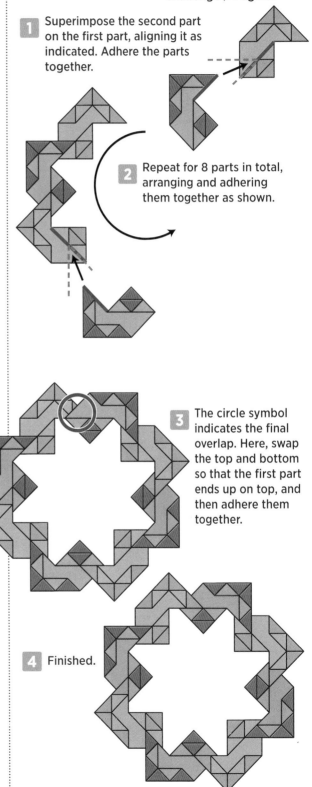

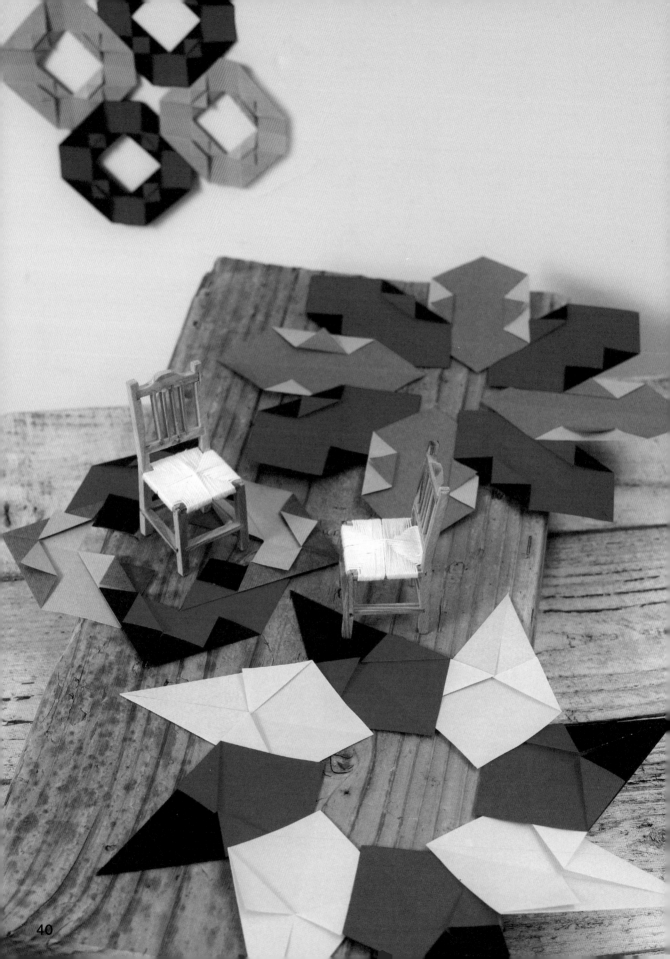

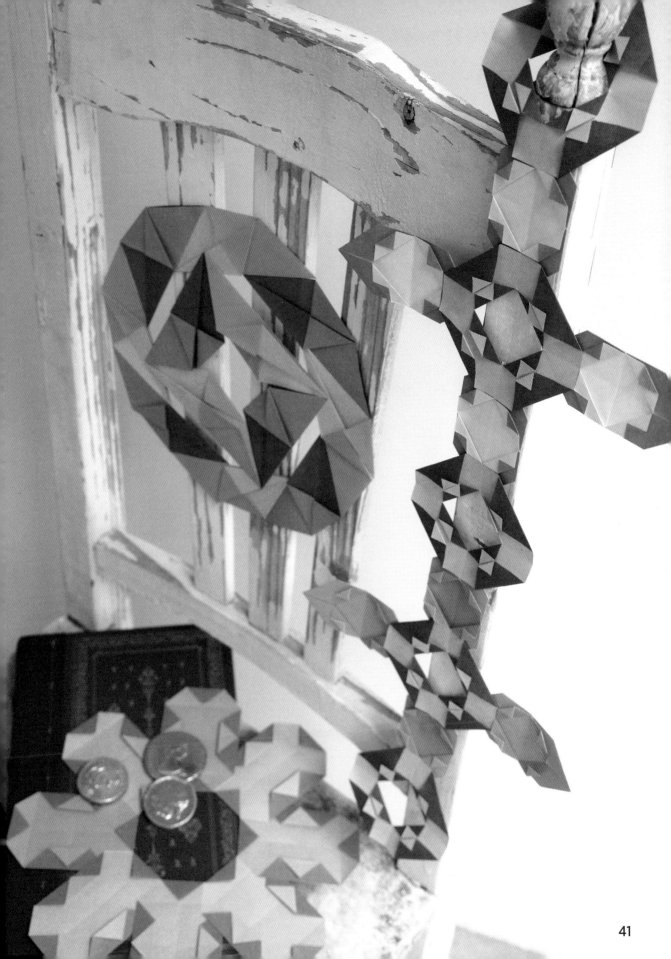

M Shape

Using the carefully made creases, fold back the corners to create the letter M. A single part has a jagged appearance, but when several are arranged in a circle, they resemble a cheerful blossom.

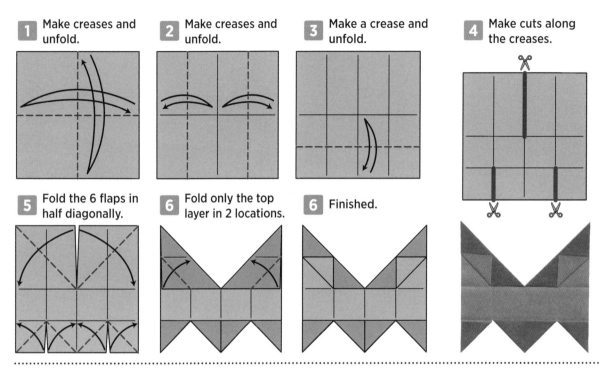

1 Make creases and unfold.

2 Make creases and unfold.

3 Make a crease and unfold.

4 Make cuts along the creases.

5 Fold the 6 flaps in half diagonally.

6 Fold only the top layer in 2 locations.

6 Finished.

Boomerang

Repeatedly making folds increases the thickness with layers of paper. Use a bone folder or the bowl of a spoon to firmly press each crease. After completing the part, it is recommended to press it under a heavy book for a while before using it.

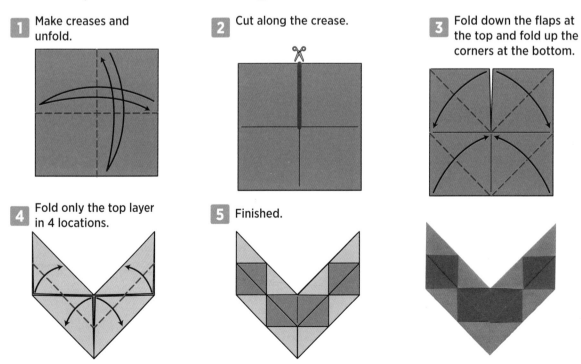

1 Make creases and unfold.

2 Cut along the crease.

3 Fold down the flaps at the top and fold up the corners at the bottom.

4 Fold only the top layer in 4 locations.

5 Finished.

Combine 4 M Shape parts to create a shape.

Method
▶ *Page 44*

×4

Combine 8 M Shape parts to create a shape.

Method
▶ *Page 44*

×8

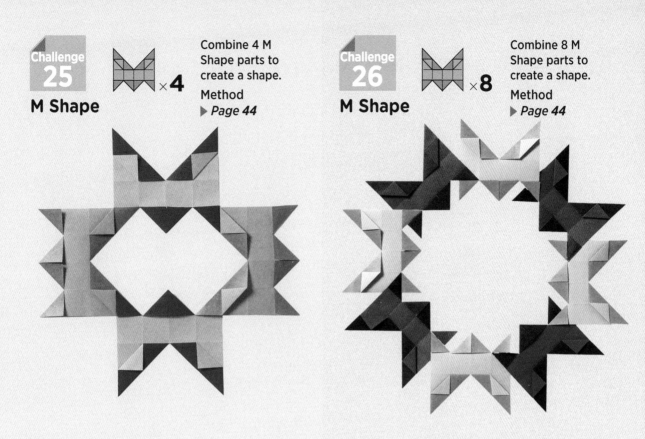

There are many other ways to assemble these parts in addition to the examples set forth in these challenges. Use your imagination to devise new configurations and design your own compositions.

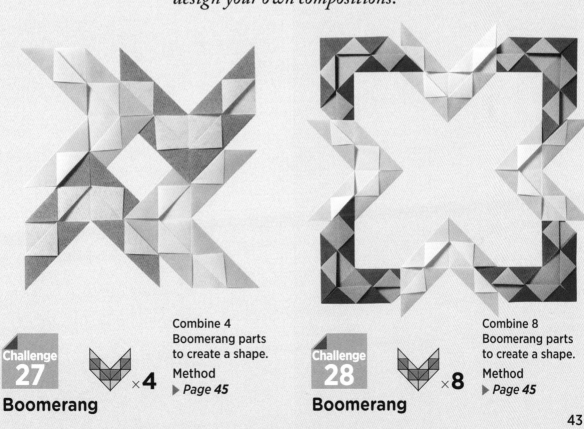

×4

Combine 4 Boomerang parts to create a shape.

Method
▶ *Page 45*

×8

Combine 8 Boomerang parts to create a shape.

Method
▶ *Page 45*

Methods for
M Shape Challenges

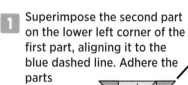

Method 25 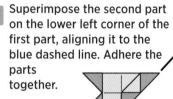 ×**4**

Challenge ▶ *Page 43*

1 Superimpose the second part on the lower left corner of the first part, aligning it to the blue dashed line. Adhere the parts together.

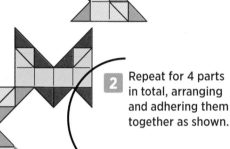

2 Repeat for 4 parts in total, arranging and adhering them together as shown.

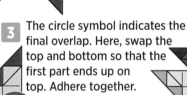

3 The circle symbol indicates the final overlap. Here, swap the top and bottom so that the first part ends up on top. Adhere together.

4 Finished.

Method 26 ×**8**

Challenge ▶ *Page 43*

1 Superimpose the second part on the lower left area of the first part, aligning it as indicated. Adhere the parts together.

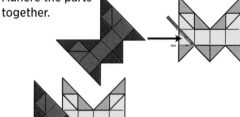

2 Repeat for 8 parts in total, arranging and adhering them together as shown.

3 The circle symbol indicates the final overlap. Here, swap the top and bottom so that the first part ends up on top. Adhere them together.

4 Finished.

Methods for
Boomerang Challenges

Challenge ▶ *Page 43*

1 Superimpose the second part on the left area of the first part, aligning it to the blue dashed line. Adhere the parts together.

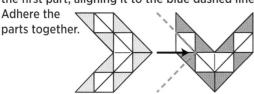

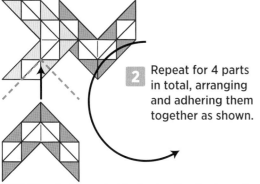

2 Repeat for 4 parts in total, arranging and adhering them together as shown.

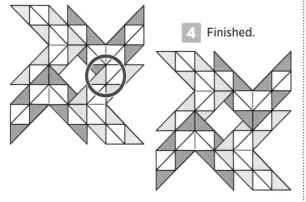

3 The circle symbol indicates the final overlap. Here, swap the top and bottom so that the first part ends up on top. Adhere them together.

4 Finished.

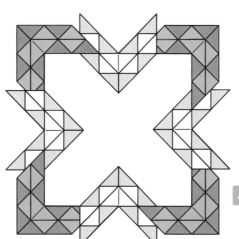

Challenge ▶ *Page 43*

1 Superimpose the second part on the upper left area of the first part, aligning it to the blue dashed line. Adhere the parts together.

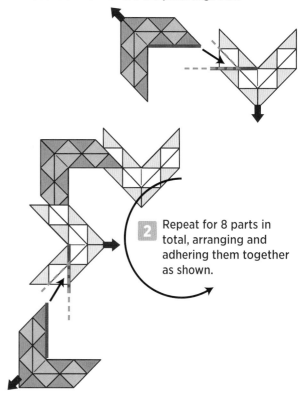

2 Repeat for 8 parts in total, arranging and adhering them together as shown.

3 The circle symbol indicates the final overlap. Here, swap the top and bottom so that the first part ends up on top. Adhere them together.

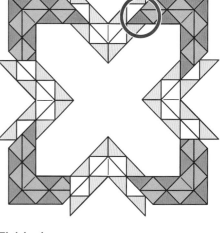

4 Finished.

Arrowhead

In step 3, it might seem unclear where to align the corner for folding. However, if you look ahead at the diagram for step 4 to confirm the position, you can finish without mistakes.

1 Fold the paper in half.

2 Fold only the top layer, aligning the cut edge to the folded edge.

3 Fold only the top layer, aligning the ☆ corner to the ★ point near the center. It's easier if you first look ahead to step 4.

4 Finished.

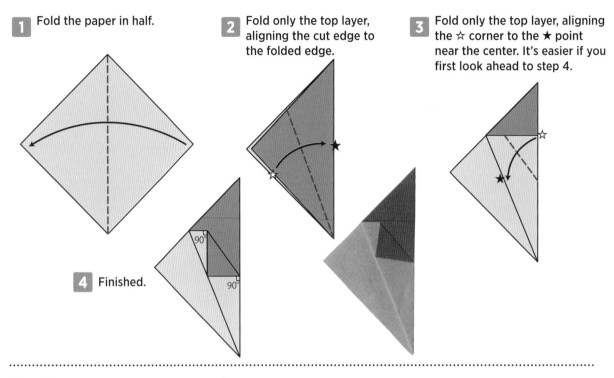

Feather

This part has an asymmetrical shape like a feather. When assembled in a circular pattern, it results in a creation that looks like a large windmill.

1 Fold the paper in half.

2 Fold only the top layer, aligning the cut edge to the folded edge.

3 Fold only single layers, aligning the ☆ edges to the ★ point near the center.

4 Finished.

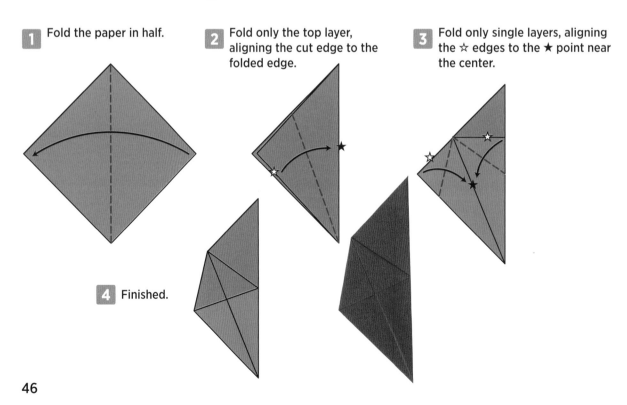

46

Challenge
29
Arrowhead ×**4**

Combine 4
Arrowhead parts
to create a shape.
Method
▶ *Page 48*

Challenge
30
Arrowhead ×**8**

Combine 8
Arrowhead parts
to create a shape.
Method
▶ *Page 48*

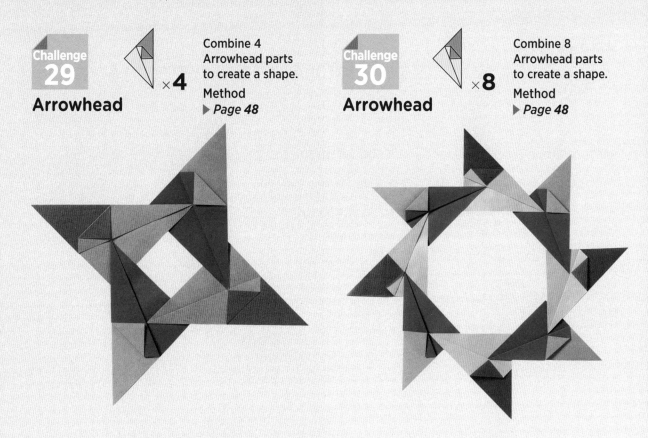

Looking at the vibrant colors makes my heart flutter.

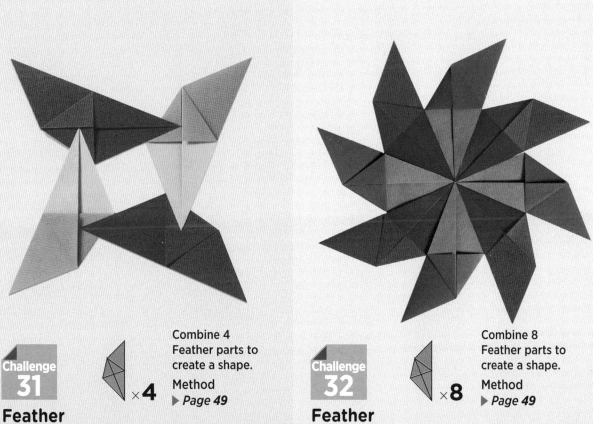

Challenge
31
Feather ×**4**

Combine 4
Feather parts to
create a shape.
Method
▶ *Page 49*

Challenge
32
Feather ×**8**

Combine 8
Feather parts to
create a shape.
Method
▶ *Page 49*

Methods for
Arrowhead Challenges

Method 29 ×4

Challenge ▶ *Page 47*

1 Superimpose the second part on the lower left area of the first part, aligning it as indicated. Adhere the parts together.

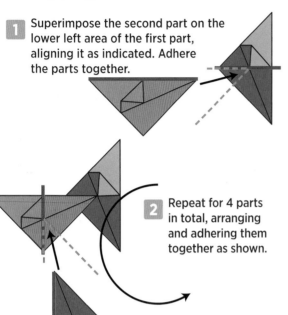

2 Repeat for 4 parts in total, arranging and adhering them together as shown.

3 The circle symbol indicates the final overlap. Here, swap the top and bottom so that the first part ends up on top, and then adhere them together.

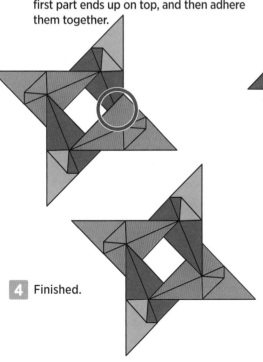

4 Finished.

Method 30 ×8

Challenge ▶ *Page 47*

1 Superimpose the second part on the lower left area of the first part, aligning it as indicated. Adhere the parts together.

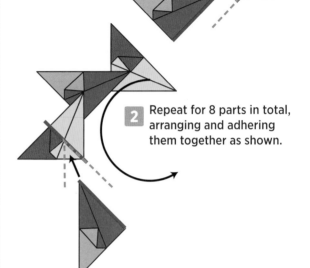

2 Repeat for 8 parts in total, arranging and adhering them together as shown.

3 The circle symbol indicates the final overlap. Here, swap the top and bottom so that the first part ends up on top, and then adhere together.

4 Finished.

Feather Challenges

Method 31 ×**4**

Challenge ▶ *Page 47*

Method 32 ×**8**

Challenge ▶ *Page 47*

1 Superimpose the second part on the left area of the first part, aligning it as indicated. Adhere the parts together.

1 Align the edges of 2 Feather parts as indicated, and tape them together on the back.

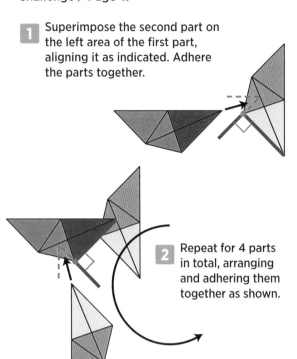

2 Repeat for 4 parts in total, arranging and adhering them together as shown.

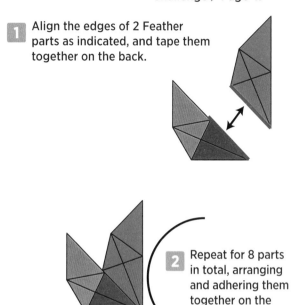

2 Repeat for 8 parts in total, arranging and adhering them together on the back as shown.

3 The circle symbol indicates the final overlap. Here, swap the top and bottom so that the first part ends up on top, and then adhere them together.

3 Finished.

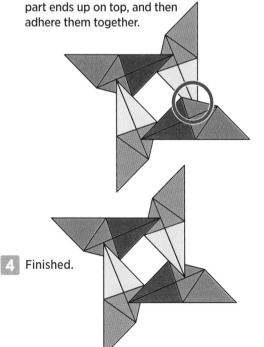

4 Finished.

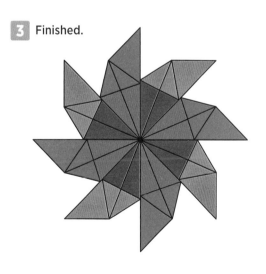

Drum

This part looks beautiful when arranged in a circle, but when placed in series vertically or horizontally, they can be used to represent columns or walls of buildings. They are used in this book for advanced projects like the Fairy-Tale Castle (page 74) and the Carp Streamer (page 93).

1 Make creases and unfold.

2 Make creases and unfold.

3 Make cuts along the creases.

4 Fold the left and right flaps in half horizontally.

5 Fold in the 4 flaps.

6 Finished.

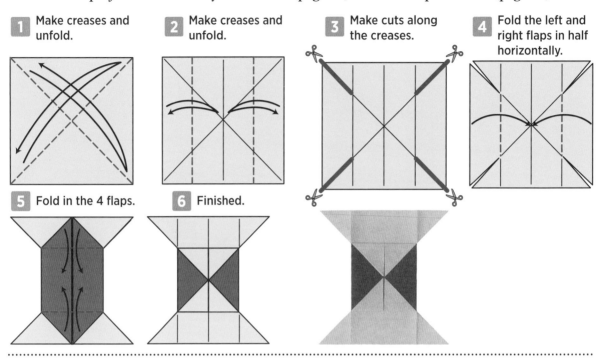

Plus Symbol

For the cuts in step 6, start from the center of the paper and carefully cut outward with the tips of the scissors. Because there are many folds, press the part under a heavy book to flatten it before use.

1 Make creases and unfold.

2 Make creases and unfold.

3 Make creases and unfold.

4 Fold the paper in half.

5 Cut as indicated through both layers, then unfold.

6 Cut along the indicated creases.

7 Valley fold flaps in 12 locations.

8 Finished.

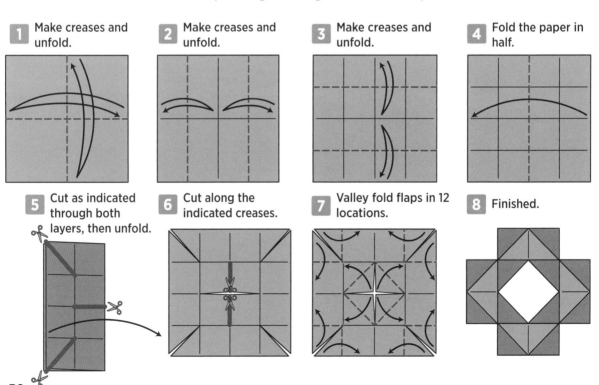

50

×**4**

Combine 4 Drum parts to create a shape.
Method
▶ *Page 52*

 ×**8**

Combine 8 Drum parts to create a shape.
Method
▶ *Page 52*

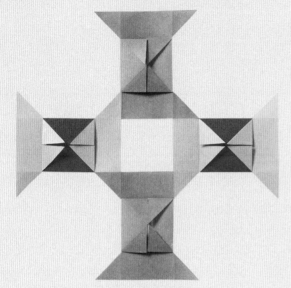

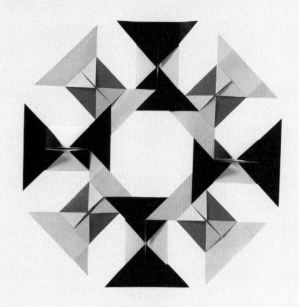

It's also fun to have several people make parts and assemble them into one work.

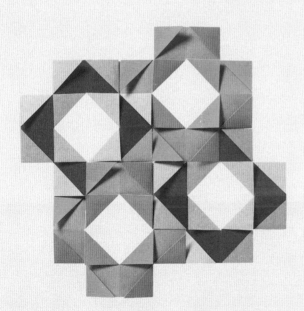

 Challenge 35 **Plus Symbol**

 ×**4**

Combine 4 Plus Symbol parts to create a shape.
Method
▶ *Page 53*

Challenge 36 **Plus Symbol**

 ×**8**

Combine 8 Plus Symbol parts to create a shape.
Method
▶ *Page 53*

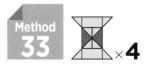

Challenge ▶ *Page 51*

Challenge ▶ *Page 51*

1 Superimpose the second part on the lower left corner of the first part, aligning it to the blue dashed line. Adhere the parts together.

1 Superimpose the second part on the lower left corner of the first part, aligning it to the blue dashed line. Adhere the parts together.

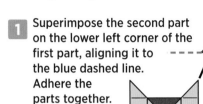

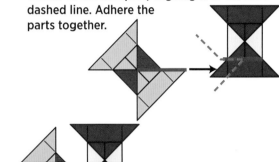

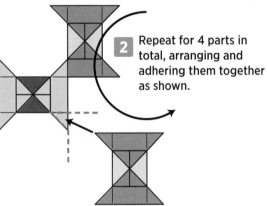

2 Repeat for 4 parts in total, arranging and adhering them together as shown.

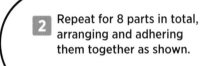

2 Repeat for 8 parts in total, arranging and adhering them together as shown.

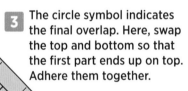

3 The circle symbol indicates the final overlap. Here, swap the top and bottom so that the first part ends up on top. Adhere them together.

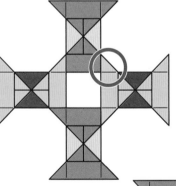

3 The circle symbol indicates the final overlap. Here, swap the top and bottom so that the first part ends up on top. Adhere them together.

4 Finished.

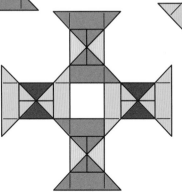

4 Finished.

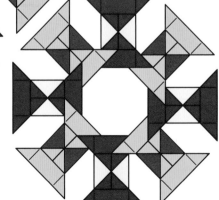

Method 35 ×**4**

Challenge ▶ *Page 51*

Method 36 ×**8**

Challenge ▶ *Page 51*

1 Superimpose the second part on the lower left area of the first part, aligning it to the blue dashed line. Adhere the parts together.

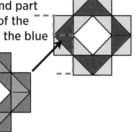

1 Superimpose the second part on the lower left area of the first part, aligning it as indicated. Adhere the parts together.

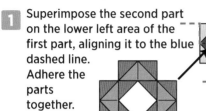

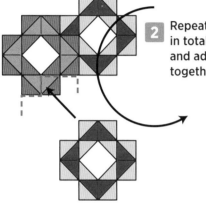

2 Repeat for 4 parts in total, arranging and adhering them together as shown.

2 Repeat for 8 parts in total, arranging and adhering them together as shown.

3 The circle symbol indicates the final overlap. Here, swap the top and bottom so the first part ends up on top. Adhere them together.

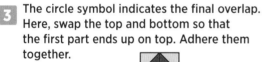

3 The circle symbol indicates the final overlap. Here, swap the top and bottom so that the first part ends up on top. Adhere them together.

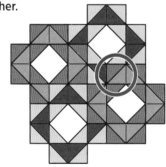

4 Finished.

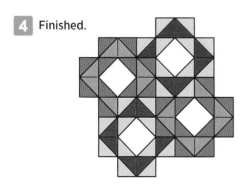

4 Finished.

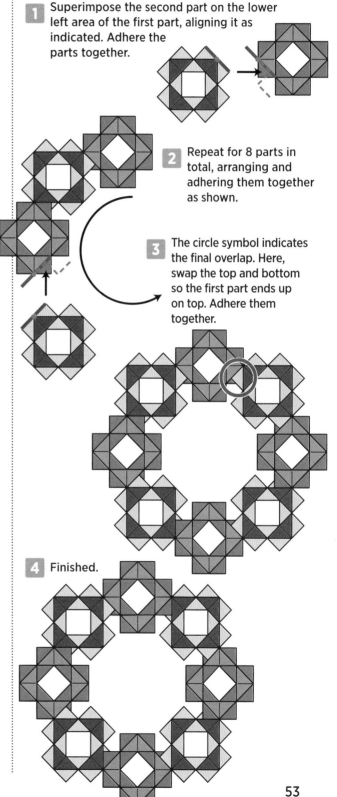

Necktie

Before folding the left corner to the right with a valley fold in step 3, look ahead to step 4 to confirm which crease to align the top edge of the flap with.

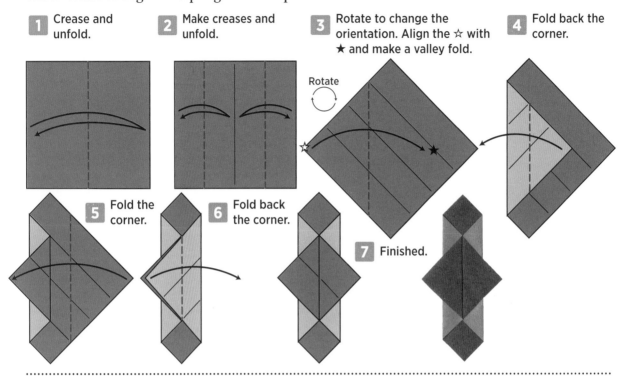

1 Crease and unfold.

2 Make creases and unfold.

3 Rotate to change the orientation. Align the ☆ with ★ and make a valley fold.

Rotate

4 Fold back the corner.

5 Fold the corner.

6 Fold back the corner.

7 Finished.

Oval Coin

When folding at step 2, if the entire paper is not perfectly square, the folded parts may overlap slightly. But because you will unfold the top and bottom flaps after this step, this is not a concern.

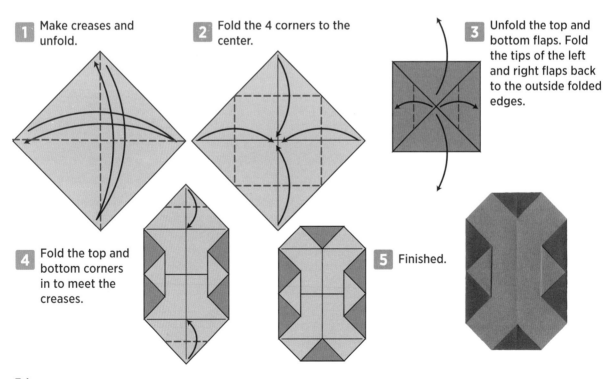

1 Make creases and unfold.

2 Fold the 4 corners to the center.

3 Unfold the top and bottom flaps. Fold the tips of the left and right flaps back to the outside folded edges.

4 Fold the top and bottom corners in to meet the creases.

5 Finished.

×4

Combine 4 Necktie parts to create a shape.
Method
▶ *Page 56*

×8

Combine 8 Necktie parts to create a shape.
Method
▶ *Page 56*

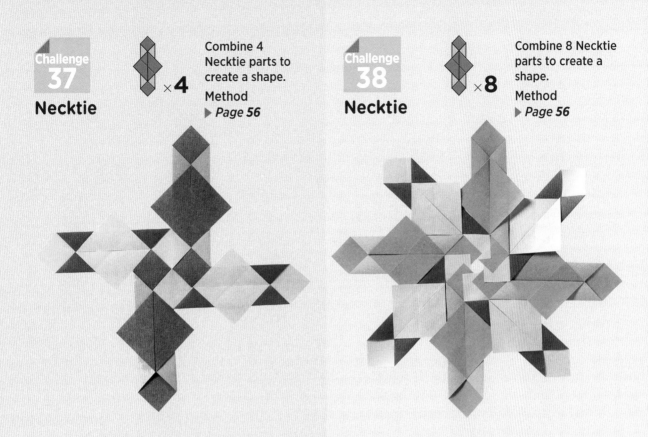

Besides affixing them to a wall or hanging them with thread, try using these assemblies as placemats or coasters.

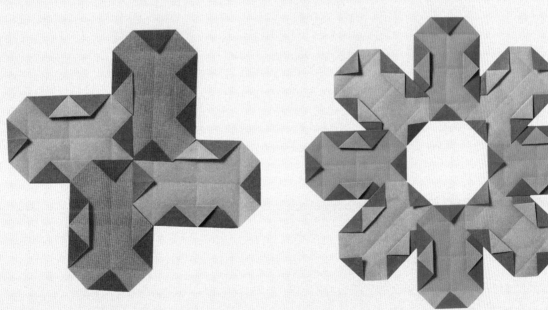

×4

Combine 4 Oval Coin parts to create a shape.
Method
▶ *Page 57*

Oval Coin

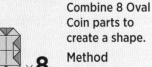

×8

Combine 8 Oval Coin parts to create a shape.
Method
▶ *Page 57*

Oval Coin

Method 37 ×4

Challenge ▶ Page 55

1 Superimpose the second part on the lower left area of the first part, aligning it to the blue dashed line. Adhere the parts together.

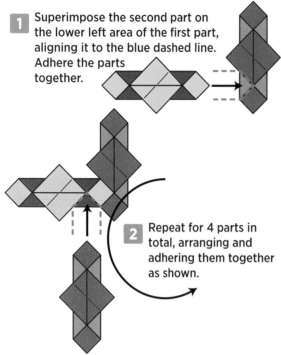

2 Repeat for 4 parts in total, arranging and adhering them together as shown.

3 The circle symbol indicates the final overlap. Here, swap the top and bottom so that the first part ends up on top. Adhere them together.

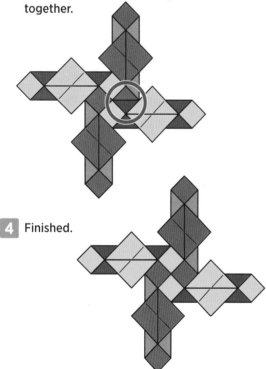

4 Finished.

Method 38 ×8

Challenge ▶ Page 55

1 Superimpose the second part on the lower left area of the first part, aligning it to the blue dashed line. Adhere the parts together.

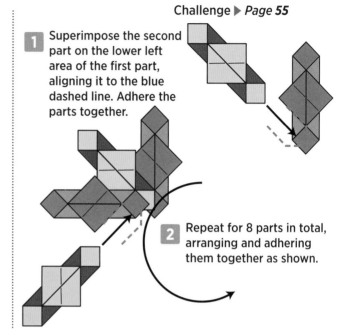

2 Repeat for 8 parts in total, arranging and adhering them together as shown.

3 The circle symbol indicates the final overlap. Here, swap the top and bottom so that the first part ends up on top. Adhere them together.

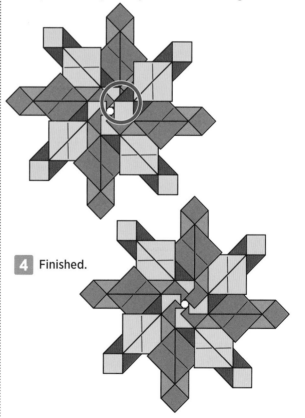

4 Finished.

Method 39 ×**4**

Challenge ▶ *Page 55*

1 Superimpose the second part on the lower left area of the first part, aligning it to the blue dashed line. Adhere the parts together.

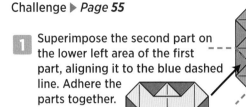

2 Repeat for 4 parts in total, arranging and adhering them together as shown.

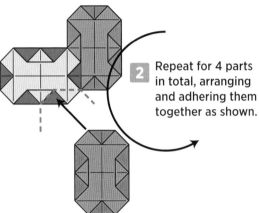

3 The circle symbol indicates the final overlap. Here, swap the top and bottom so that the first part ends up on top. Adhere them together.

4 Finished.

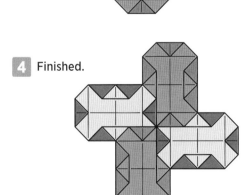

Method 40 ×**8**

Challenge ▶ *Page 55*

1 Superimpose the second part on the lower left area of the first part, aligning it as indicated. Adhere the parts together.

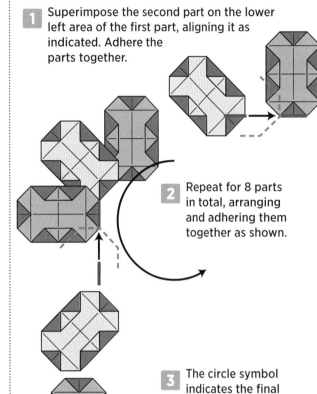

2 Repeat for 8 parts in total, arranging and adhering them together as shown.

3 The circle symbol indicates the final overlap. Here, swap the top and bottom so that the first part ends up on top. Adhere together.

4 Finished.

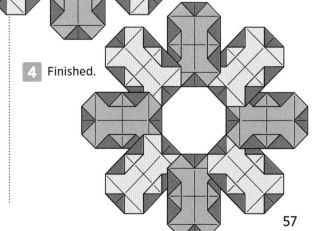

Leaf Badge

The overall shape resembles the "beginner's mark" displayed on the cars of new drivers in Japan. The small triangles that appear at step 7 give it a characteristic modular origami look.

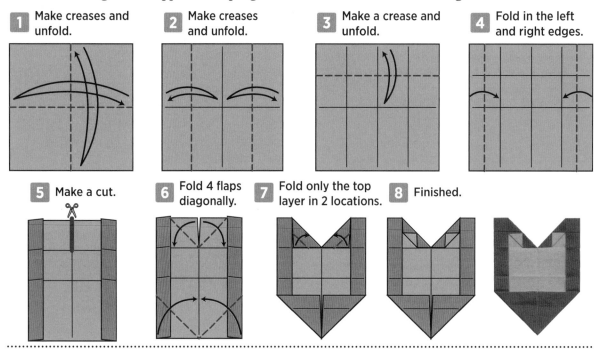

1 Make creases and unfold.

2 Make creases and unfold.

3 Make a crease and unfold.

4 Fold in the left and right edges.

5 Make a cut.

6 Fold 4 flaps diagonally.

7 Fold only the top layer in 2 locations.

8 Finished.

Gem

This part finishes with intricate geometric beauty, much like a gem. The arrangements created by combining several parts make an even more dramatic impression, making it difficult to believe they were made by hand without using a ruler.

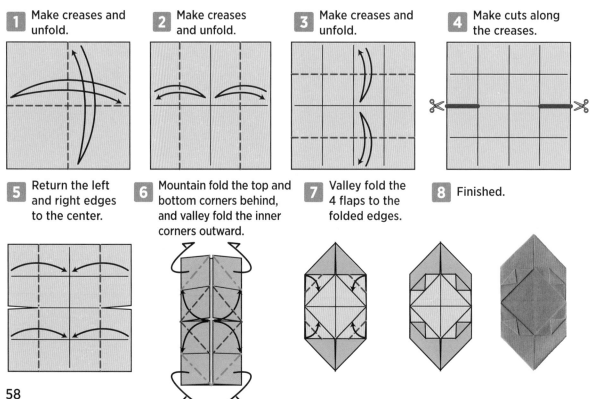

1 Make creases and unfold.

2 Make creases and unfold.

3 Make creases and unfold.

4 Make cuts along the creases.

5 Return the left and right edges to the center.

6 Mountain fold the top and bottom corners behind, and valley fold the inner corners outward.

7 Valley fold the 4 flaps to the folded edges.

8 Finished.

58

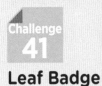 ×4

Combine 4 Leaf Badge parts to create a shape.

Method
▶ *Page 60*

 ×8

Combine 8 Leaf Badge parts to create a shape.

Method
▶ *Page 60*

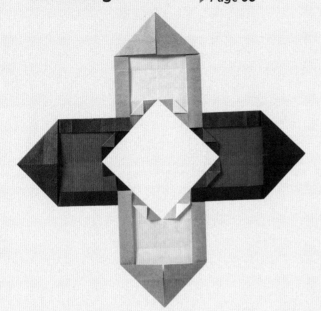

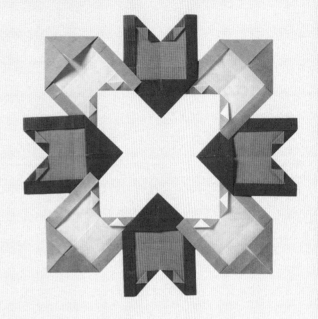

The beautiful appearance of the finished assemblies makes creating these pieces an exciting brain exercise for young and old alike.

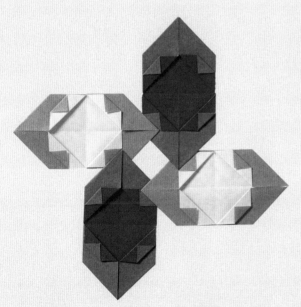

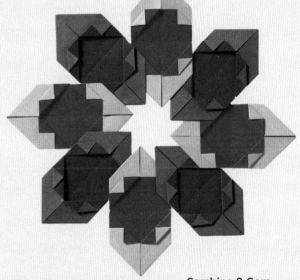

Combine 4 Gem parts to create a shape.

Method
▶ *Page 61*

Challenge 43

 ×4

Gem

Combine 8 Gem parts to create a shape.

Method
▶ *Page 61*

Challenge 44

 ×8

Gem

Method 41 ×4

Challenge ▶ *Page 59*

Method 42 ×8

Challenge ▶ *Page 59*

1 Superimpose the second part on the lower left corner of the first part, aligning it as indicated. Adhere the parts together.

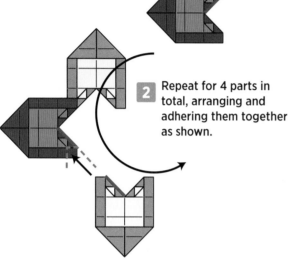

2 Repeat for 4 parts in total, arranging and adhering them together as shown.

3 The circle symbol indicates the final overlap. Here, swap the top and bottom so that the first part ends up on top. Adhere them together.

4 Finished.

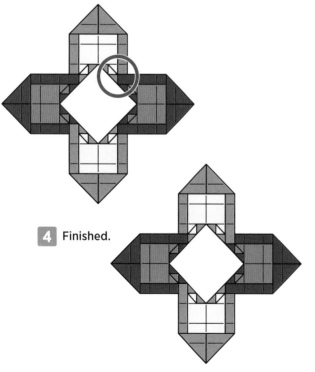

1 Superimpose the second part on the left area of the first part, aligning it as indicated. Adhere the parts together.

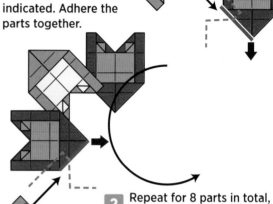

2 Repeat for 8 parts in total, arranging and adhering them together as shown.

3 The circle symbol indicates the final overlap. Here, swap the top and bottom so that the first part ends up on top. Adhere them together.

4 Finished.

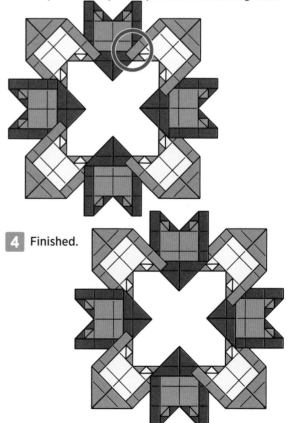

Method 43 ×**4**

Methods for
Gem Challenges

Method 44 ×**8**

Challenge ▶ *Page 59*

1 Superimpose the second part on the lower left area of the first part, aligning it as indicated. Adhere the parts together.

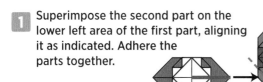

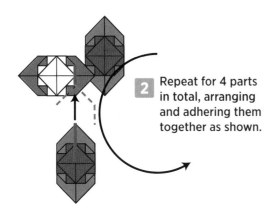

2 Repeat for 4 parts in total, arranging and adhering them together as shown.

3 The circle symbol indicates the final overlap. Here, swap the top and bottom so that the first part ends up on top. Adhere them together.

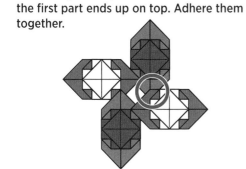

4 Finished.

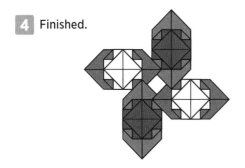

Challenge ▶ *Page 59*

1 Superimpose the second part on the lower left area of the first part, aligning it as indicated. Adhere the parts together.

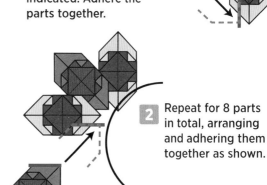

2 Repeat for 8 parts in total, arranging and adhering them together as shown.

3 The circle symbol indicates the final overlap. Here, swap the top and bottom so that the first part ends up on top. Adhere them together.

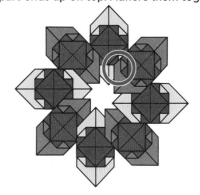

4 Finished.

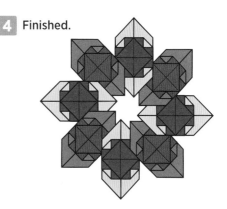

Prism

In step 9, aligning the corners precisely is the key to a clean finish. Although this part has many steps, press the creases firmly with a bone folder or the bowl of a spoon and proceed carefully.

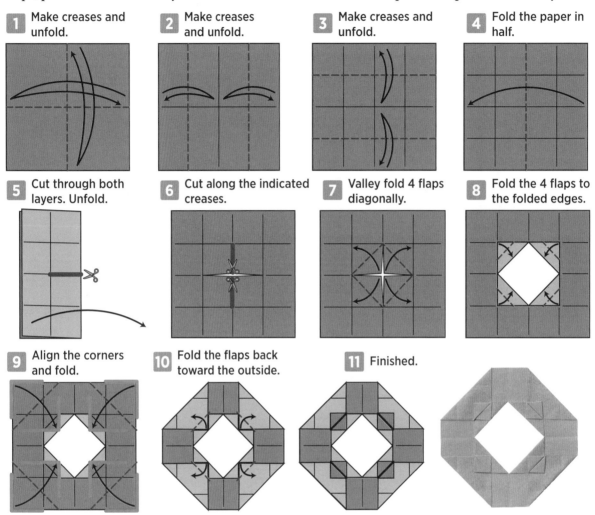

1 Make creases and unfold.

2 Make creases and unfold.

3 Make creases and unfold.

4 Fold the paper in half.

5 Cut through both layers. Unfold.

6 Cut along the indicated creases.

7 Valley fold 4 flaps diagonally.

8 Fold the 4 flaps to the folded edges.

9 Align the corners and fold.

10 Fold the flaps back toward the outside.

11 Finished.

Trapezoid

This part is very similar to Mount Fuji (page 20). When folding down the upper corner to touch the bottom edge in step 2, there's no landmark to reference, but bring the corner to the center point, where the spans on both sides of the bottom edge are equal.

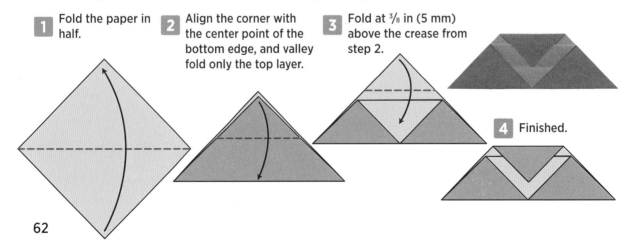

1 Fold the paper in half.

2 Align the corner with the center point of the bottom edge, and valley fold only the top layer.

3 Fold at ³⁄₈ in (5 mm) above the crease from step 2.

4 Finished.

Challenge 45

Prism

Combine 4 Prism parts to create a shape.

Method
▶ *Page 64*

Challenge 46

Prism

Combine 8 Prism parts to create a shape.

Method
▶ *Page 64*

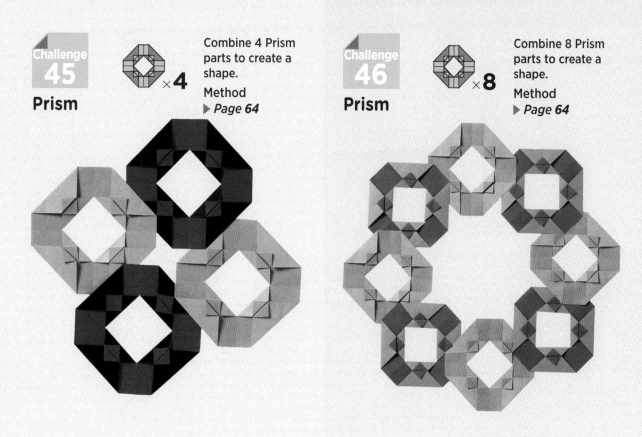

You have now finished learning how to fold all 24 types of parts!

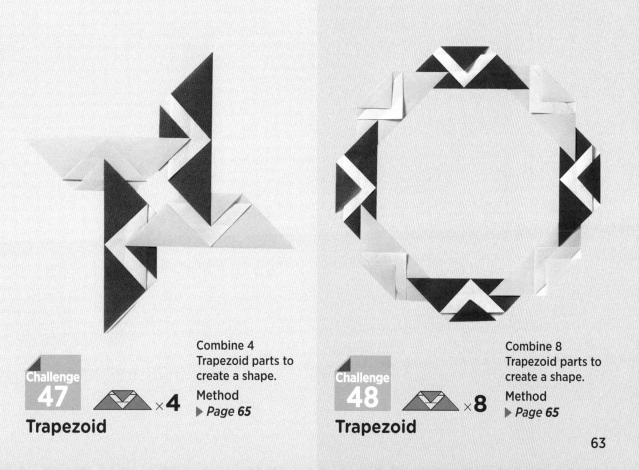

Challenge 47

Trapezoid

Combine 4 Trapezoid parts to create a shape.

Method
▶ *Page 65*

Challenge 48

Trapezoid

Combine 8 Trapezoid parts to create a shape.

Method
▶ *Page 65*

Methods for
Prism Challenges

  ×**4**

Method 45

Challenge ▶ *Page 63*

  ×**8**

Method 46

Challenge ▶ *Page 63*

1 Superimpose the second part on the lower left area of the first part, aligning it to the blue dashed line. Adhere the parts together.

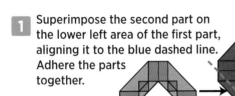

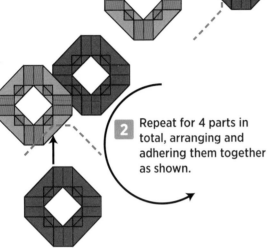

2 Repeat for 4 parts in total, arranging and adhering them together as shown.

1 Superimpose the second part on the lower left area of the first part, aligning it to the blue dashed line. Adhere the parts together.

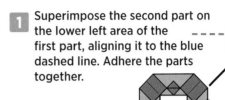

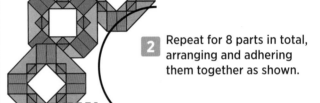

2 Repeat for 8 parts in total, arranging and adhering them together as shown.

3 The circle symbol indicates the final overlap. Here, swap the top and bottom so that the first part ends up on top. Adhere them together.

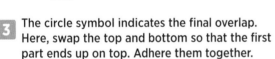

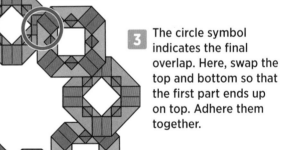

3 The circle symbol indicates the final overlap. Here, swap the top and bottom so that the first part ends up on top. Adhere them together.

4 Finished.

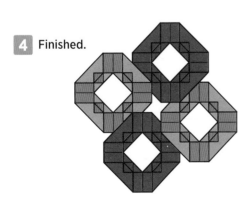

4 Finished.

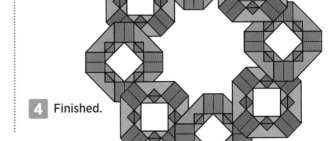

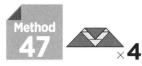

Methods for
Trapezoid Challenges

Method 47 ×4

Challenge ▶ *Page 63*

1 Superimpose the second part on the lower left area of the first part, aligning it to the blue dashed line. Adhere the parts together.

2 Repeat for 4 parts in total, arranging and adhering them together as shown.

3 The circle symbol indicates the final overlap. Here, swap the top and bottom so that the first part ends up on top. Adhere them together.

4 Finished.

Method 48 ×8

Challenge ▶ *Page 63*

1 Superimpose the second part on the lower left corner of the first part, aligning it as indicated. Adhere the parts together.

2 Repeat for 8 parts in total, arranging and adhering them together as shown.

3 The circle symbol indicates the final overlap. Here, swap the top and bottom so that the first part ends up on top. Adhere them together.

4 Finished.

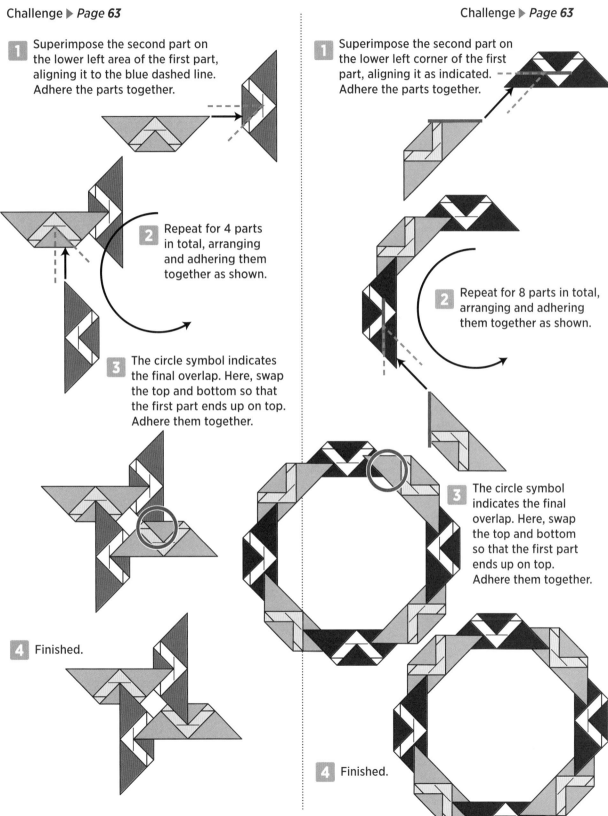

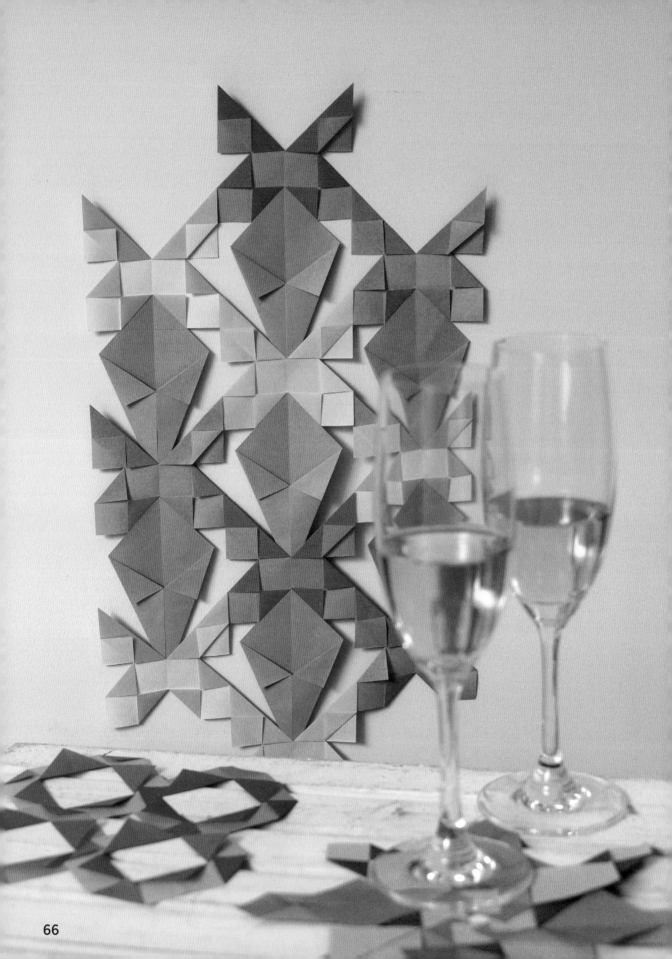

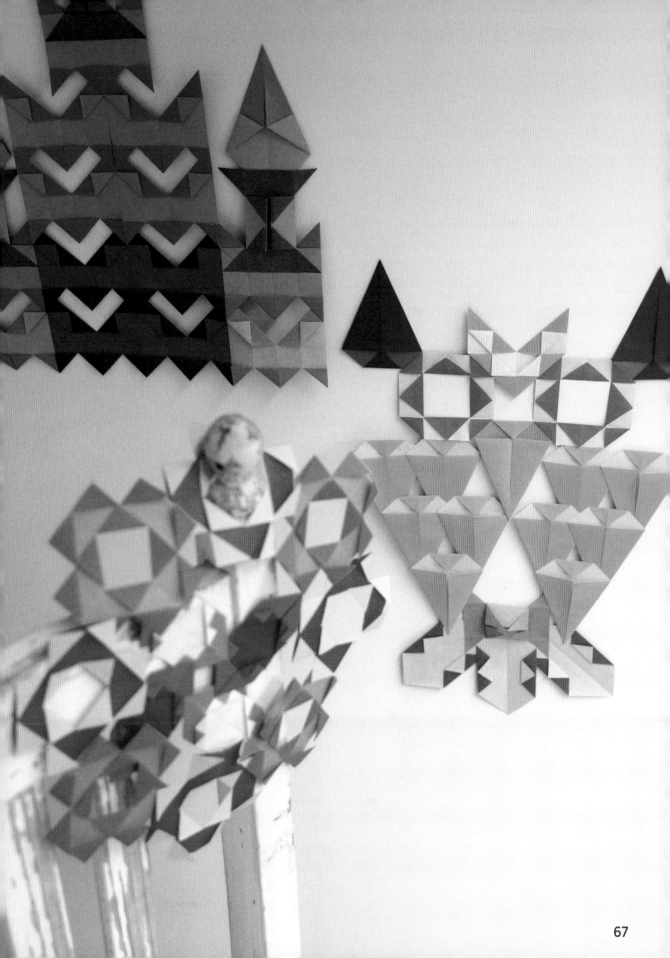

Spring

....

Seasonal
Wall Decorations

Challenge
49

Spring Flowers

Large tulips have bloomed together. Butterflies are flying around them. Create this delightful spring scene.

Origami Butterfly

Instructions ▶ *Page 69*

Tulip

Instructions ▶ *Page 70*

Stem and Leaves

Instructions
▶ *Page 71*

Flower Pot

Instructions ▶ *Page 71*

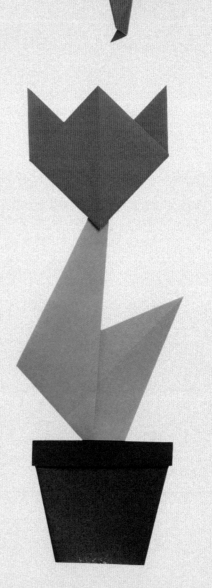

Method
49a

Challenge
▶ *Page 68*

Paper Size: Cut a 6 x 6 in (15 x 25 cm) piece of origami paper into quarters, resulting in 3 x 3 in (7.5 x 7.5 cm) squares.

Origami Butterfly

The finished piece will match the color of the paper used. Collect various colored papers and observe the impressions made by each different color.

1 Make creases and unfold.

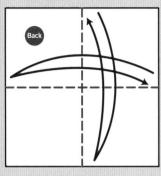

2 Make creases and unfold.

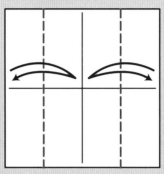

3 Make a crease and unfold.

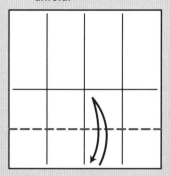

4 Make cuts along the creases.

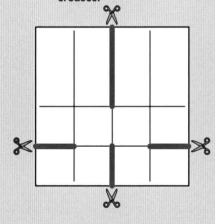

5 Fold the 8 flaps in half diagonally.

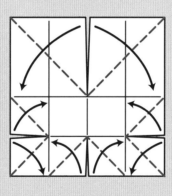

6 Fold the bottom left and right corners. Valley fold, aligning ☆ with ★.

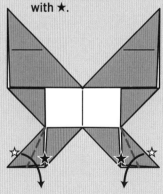

7 Flip it over.

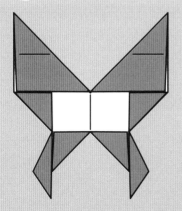

Turn over

8 Finished.

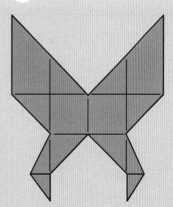

Method
49b

Challenge
▶ *Page 68*

Paper Size: Cut a 6 x 6 in (15 x 25 cm) piece of origami paper in half to make a 6 x 3 in (15 x 7.5 cm) rectangle.

Tulip

Use a rectangle cut from a 6 x 6 in (15 x 15 cm) piece of origami paper. You can make two flowers from one piece of origami paper. Try creating a circular arrangement using only the flowers.

1 Crease and unfold.

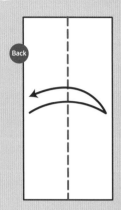

2 Crease and unfold.

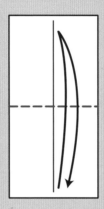

3 Crease and unfold.

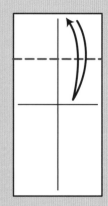

4 At the top, cut along the crease. Fold the bottom corners, aligning the ☆ edges with ★.

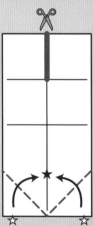

5 Fold the flaps diagonally.

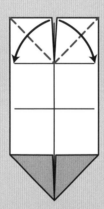

6 Fold the entire piece in half bottom to top along the existing crease.

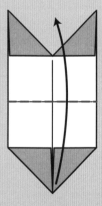

7 Fold the bottom corners to the rear.

Turn over

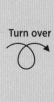

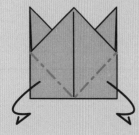

8 Finished.

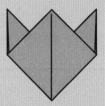

Method 49c

Challenge
▶ *Page 68*

Stem and Leaves

Use the crease to create the look of a leaf with a vein. It's a good idea to use different shades of green origami paper to create a variety of tones between leaves.

1 Cut the paper in half, yielding 2 triangles.

2 Fold, aligning ☆ with ★.

3 Fold, aligning ☆ with ★. Unfold, leaving a crease. Flip the paper left to right.

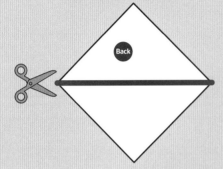
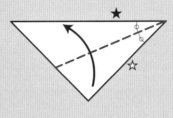
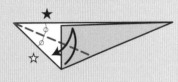

4 Fold, keeping the ☆ to ★ crease span aligned. It's easier if you look at the finished state in step 5 before starting.

Turn over

Rotate

5 Change the orientation to finish. Combine it with the Tulip.

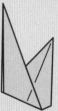

Method 49d

Challenge
▶ *Page 68*

Flower Pot

This simple origami model captures the characteristic rimmed top of the flowerpot well. This model could also be used to decorate illustrated postcards.

1 Mountain fold approximately where shown. Then, valley fold, forming a pleat.

2 Pay attention to the position and make valley folds on the left and right.

3 Flip it over.

4 Finished.

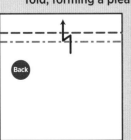
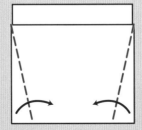
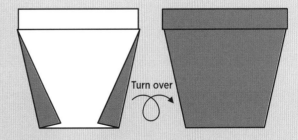

Turn over

Spring

Seasonal
Wall Decorations

Challenge 50

Thank-You Bouquet

Combine origami models of morning glories, carnations and hearts to create a lovely bouquet.

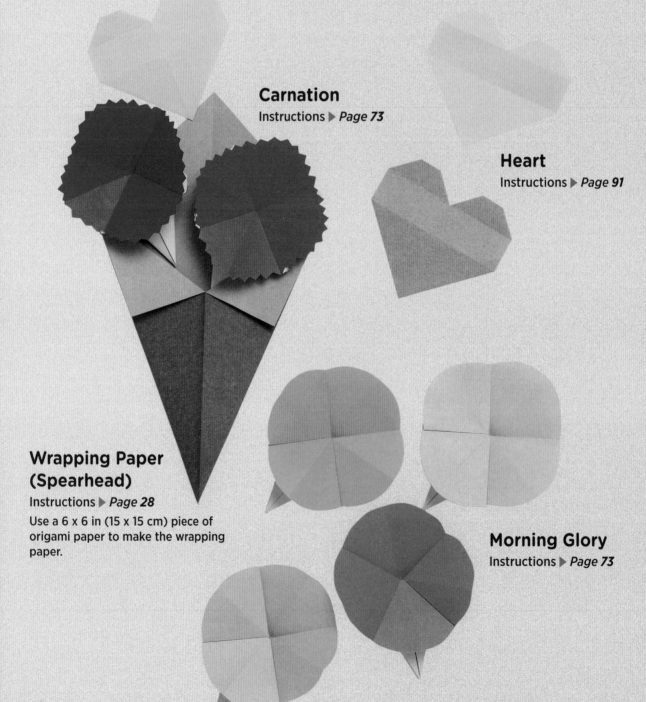

Carnation
Instructions ▶ *Page 73*

Heart
Instructions ▶ *Page 91*

Wrapping Paper (Spearhead)
Instructions ▶ *Page 28*

Use a 6 x 6 in (15 x 15 cm) piece of origami paper to make the wrapping paper.

Morning Glory
Instructions ▶ *Page 73*

Paper Size: 6 x 6 in (15 x 15 cm) square origami paper

Method 50 — Morning Glory and Carnation

Challenge
▶ *Page 72*

The folding method is practically the same for morning glories and carnations. The only difference is whether you cut the petal edges to be rounded or zigzag.

1 Make creases and unfold.

2 Fold by bringing the 3 ☆ corners to the top ★ corner, and collapse the paper.

3 Step 2 in progress.

4 The paper is collapsed.

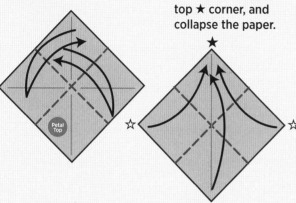

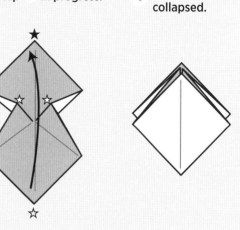

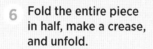

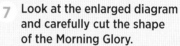

5 Align the top ☆ edges to the ★ crease. Fold the same way behind.

6 Fold the entire piece in half, make a crease, and unfold.

7 Look at the enlarged diagram and carefully cut the shape of the Morning Glory.

Cut off a small part of the corners folded in step 5. This is important!

Zoom in

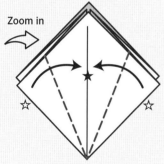

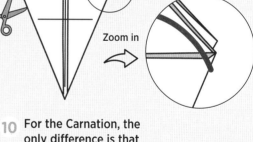

Zoom in

8 Use the crease from step 6 to open the petals. Insert your fingers into the folded paper on the left and right to open it, and fold the front part down. This will naturally form the shape.

9 The Morning Glory is completed.

10 For the Carnation, the only difference is that you cut the petal edges in a zigzag pattern in step 7. Carefully cut the shape.

11 The Carnation is completed.

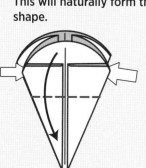

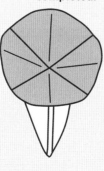

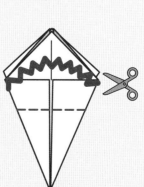

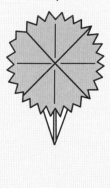

×**5**
Instructions
for Tree
▶ *Page 28*

×**3**
Instructions
for Spearhead
▶ *Page 28*

 ×**13**
Instructions
for M Shape
▶ *Page 42*

 ×**3**
Instructions
for Drum
▶ *Page 50*

Combine 24 parts from 4 different types to create a Fairy-Tale Castle.

Advanced Project

Fairy-Tale Castle
Method ▶ *Page 78*

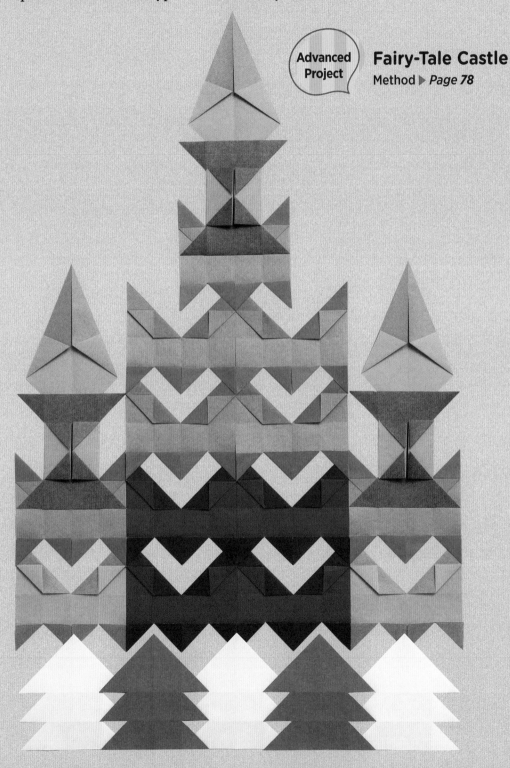

×12
Instructions
for Mini Rose
▶ *Page 16*

 ×2
Instructions
for Mount Fuji
▶ *Page 20*

 ×4
Instructions
for House
▶ *Page 24*

 ×3
Instructions
for Drum
▶ *Page 50*

Combine 21 parts from 4 different types to create the Spring Village.

Advanced Project

Spring Village
Method ▶ *Page 80*

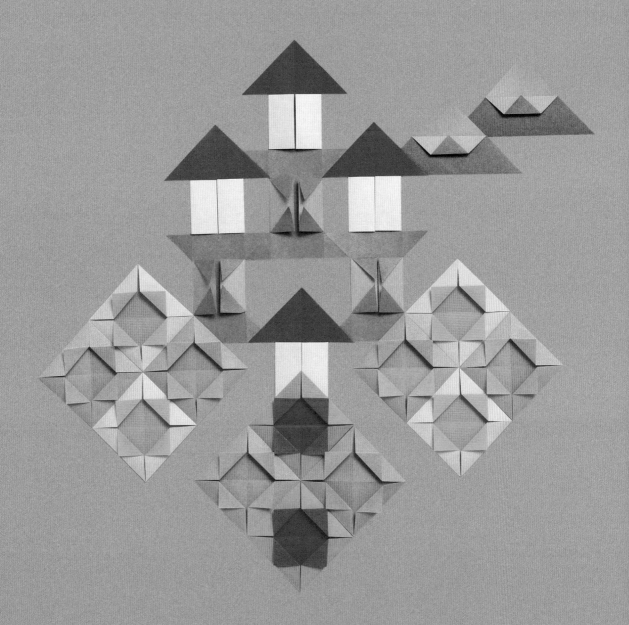

Challenge 53

 ×**8**

Instructions
for Gem
▶ *Page 58*

 ×**8**

Instructions for
Origami Butterfly
▶ *Page 69*

Combine 16 parts from 2 different types to create a Butterfly Wreath.

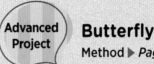

Advanced
Project

Butterfly Wreath
Method ▶ *Page 82*

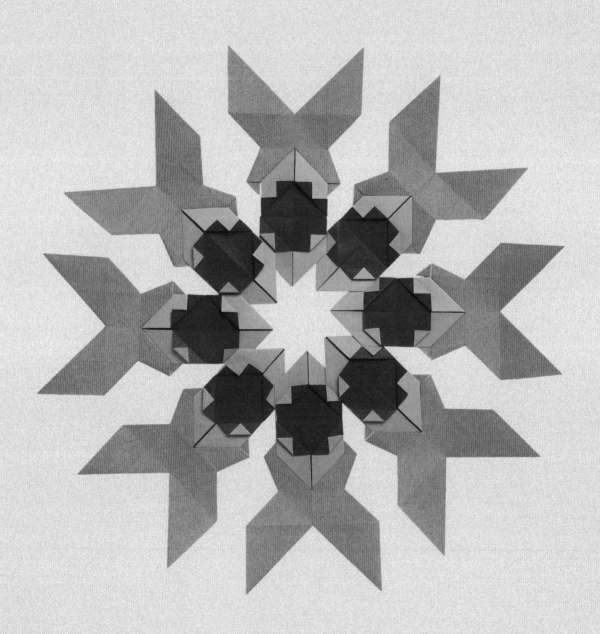

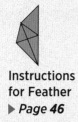

Instructions for Feather
▶ *Page 46*

Combine 12 parts of 1 type to create a Temari Wreath.

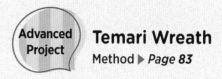

Advanced Project

Temari Wreath
Method ▶ *Page 83*

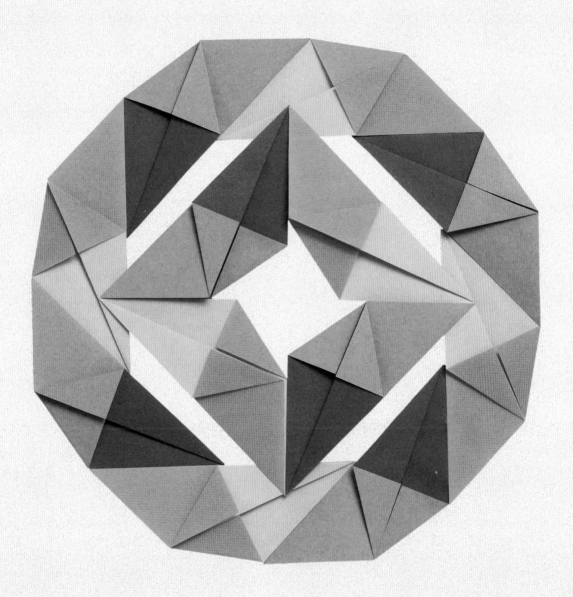

Method
51

 ×**5**
Instructions
for Tree
▶ *Page 28*

 ×**3**
Instructions
for Spearhead
▶ *Page 28*

 ×**13**
Instructions
for M Shape
▶ *Page 42*

×**3**
Instructions
for Drum
▶ *Page 50*

Advanced
Project

Fairy-Tale Castle

Challenge ▶ *Page 74*

1 Align the parts as indicated by the
blue dashed line, with the Drum
part on top. Adhere the parts
together. Make 3 sets of the same.

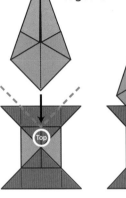

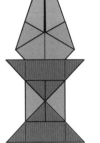 ×**3**

2 Align the edges of 2 M Shape parts as
indicated, and use tape on the back to adhere
them together. Make 4 sets of the same.

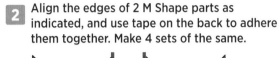

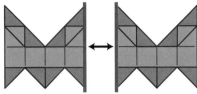

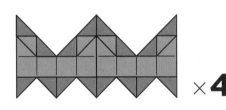 ×**4**

3 Combine the 4 sets made in step 2 in order
from bottom to top: ①, ②, ③, ④. Align the
shapes as indicated by the blue dashed line,
paying attention to their vertical alignment.

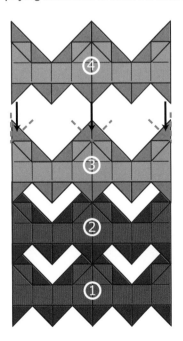

4 Add 5 M Shape parts to the step-3 assembly,
aligning them as indicated by the blue dashed
line. Use tape on the back to adhere them.

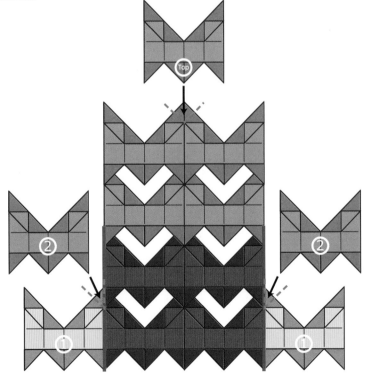

5 Place 2 Tree parts side by side, aligning the shapes as indicated by the blue dashed line, and adhere them together. Pay attention to the overlapping.

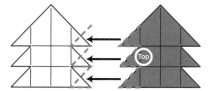

6 Place 3 more Tree parts side by side, and adhere them together. Pay attention to the overlapping.

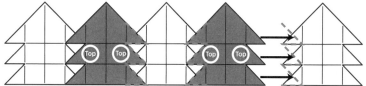

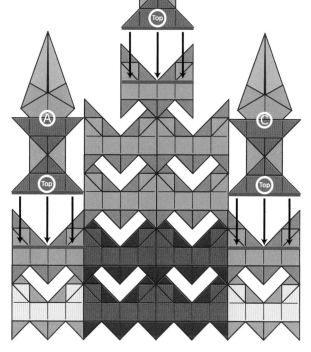

7 The 3 sets made in step 1 will form the pointed roofs of the castle. Superimpose each of A, B and C, align the shapes with the guide lines, and adhere them together. Pay attention to the overlaps.

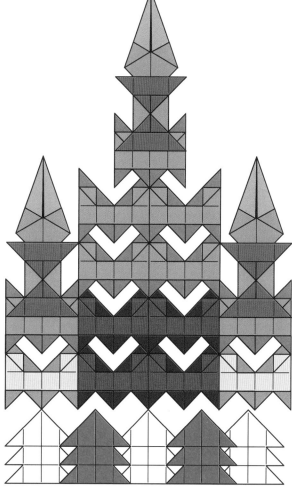

8 Place the horizontal arrangement of trees made in step 5 below the castle. Finished.

Method 52

 ×**12**

Instructions for Mini Rose
▶ *Page 16*

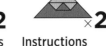 ×**2**

Instructions for Mount Fuji
▶ *Page 20*

×**4**

Instructions for House
▶ *Page 24*

 ×**3**

Instructions for Drum
▶ *Page 50*

Advanced Project

Spring Village

Challenge ▶ *Page 75*

1 Align the edges of 4 Mini Rose parts as indicated by the reference lines. Use tape on the back to adhere them together. Make 3 sets of the same.

2 Align the edges of House and Drum parts as indicated by the reference lines. Use tape on the back to adhere them together. Make 3 sets of the same.

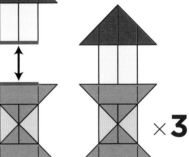

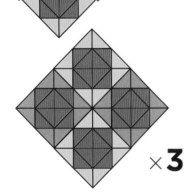

×**3**

×**3**

3 Align the edges of the 3 sets from step 2 as indicated by the reference lines. Use tape on the back to adhere them together.

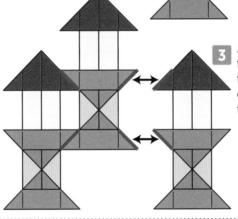

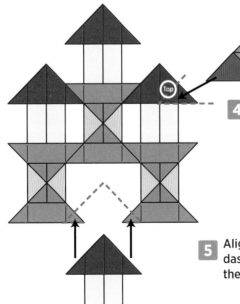

4 Align the shapes of 2 Mount Fuji parts as indicated by the blue dashed line and adhere them together. Then, position them so that the assembly from step 3 is superimposed. Align the shapes as indicated by the blue dashed line, and adhere them together.

5 Align the shapes as indicated by the blue dashed line, and adhere them together so that the bottommost House part superimposes.

6 Align the shapes as indicated by the blue dashed lines, and adhere the 3 sets from step 1 superimposed on the step-5 assembly.

7 Finished.

Method 53

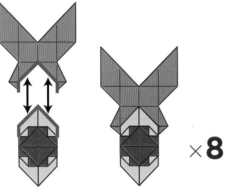

×**8**

Instructions for Gem
▶ *Page 58*

×**8**

Instructions for Origami Butterfly
▶ *Page 69*

Advanced Project

Butterfly Wreath

Challenge ▶ *Page 76*

1 Align the edges of the Gem parts and Origami Butterflies as indicated by the reference line. Use tape on the back to adhere them together. Make 8 sets of the same.

×**8**

2 Place the 8 sets from step 1 in a circular arrangement. Place the second set on the bottom left area of the first set, align the shapes as indicated by the blue dashed line, and adhere them together.

3 Repeat for 8 sets in total, arranging and adhering them together as shown.

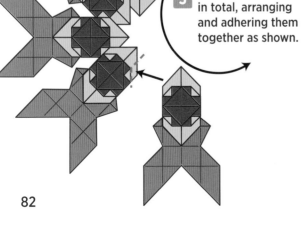

4 The oval symbol indicates the final overlap. Here, swap the top and bottom so that the first set ends up on top. Adhere them together.

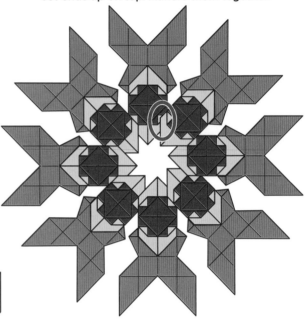

5 Finished.

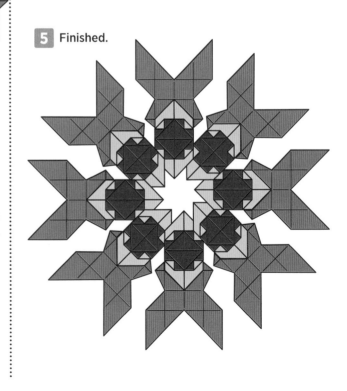

Method 54

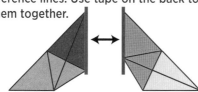 ×**12**

Instructions for Feather ▶ *Page 46*

Advanced Project

Temari Wreath

Challenge ▶ *Page 77*

1 Align the edges of the Feather parts as indicated by the reference lines. Use tape on the back to adhere them together.

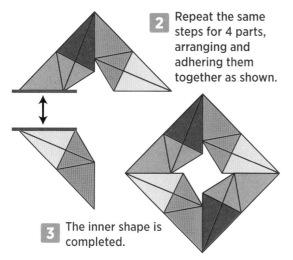

2 Repeat the same steps for 4 parts, arranging and adhering them together as shown.

3 The inner shape is completed.

4 Create the outer shape. Align the edges of the Feather parts as indicated by the reference lines. Use tape on the back to adhere them together.

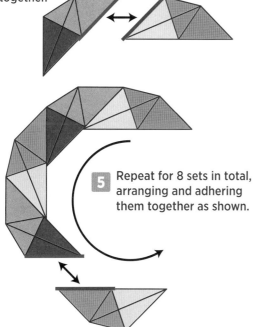

5 Repeat for 8 sets in total, arranging and adhering them together as shown.

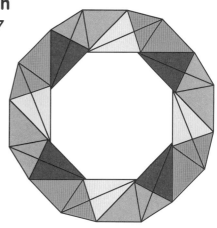

6 The outer shape is completed.

7 Align the shapes as indicated by the blue dashed line, and adhere the inner shape (step 3) superimposed on the outer shape (step 6).

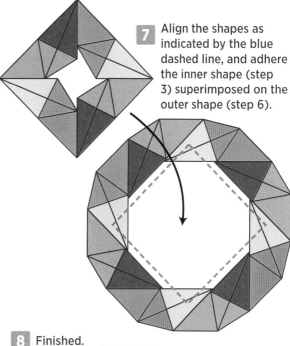

8 Finished.

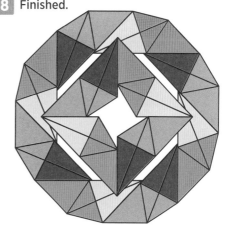

Challenge 55

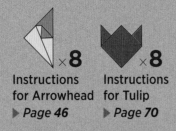

×8

Instructions for Arrowhead
▶ *Page 46*

×8

Instructions for Tulip
▶ *Page 70*

Combine 16 parts from 2 different types to create a Tulip Wreath.

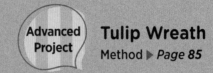

Advanced Project

Tulip Wreath

Method ▶ *Page 85*

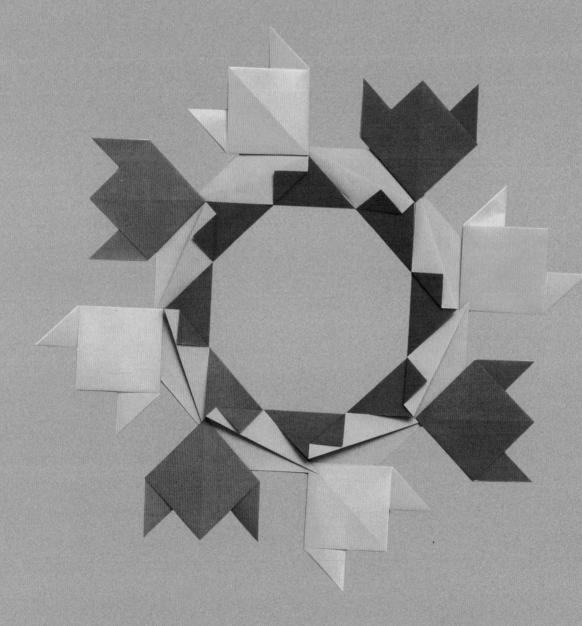

Method 55

×**8**
Instructions
for Arrowhead
▶ *Page 46*

×**8**
Instructions
for Tulip
▶ *Page 70*

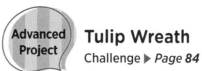

Advanced Project

Tulip Wreath

Challenge ▶ *Page 84*

1 Align the edges of the Arrowhead parts as indicated by the reference lines. Use tape on the back to adhere them together.

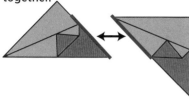

2 Repeat the same steps for 8 parts, adhering them together as shown.

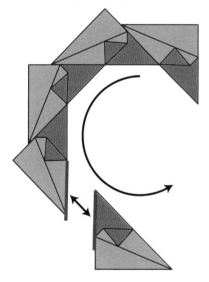

3 The inner shape is completed.

4 Align the shapes as indicated by the blue dashed lines, and adhere 8 Tulips superimposed on the inner shape (step 3).

5 Finished.

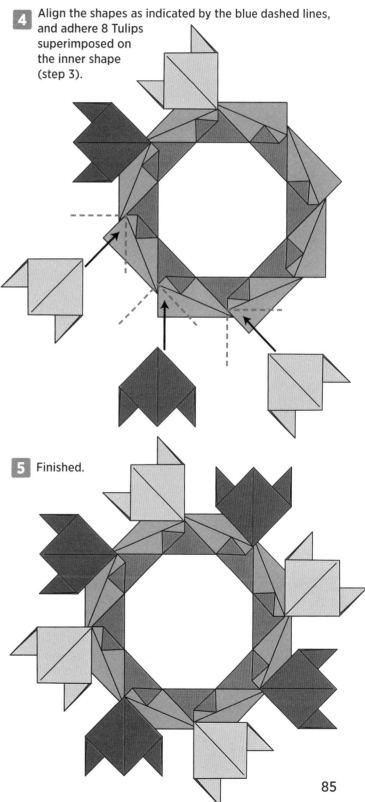

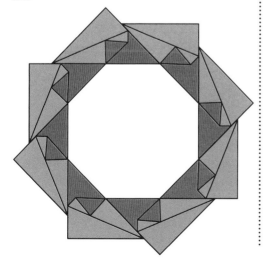

Summer

···

Seasonal
Wall Decorations

Challenge 56

Fish & Cicada

Make lots of Fish and Cicadas to decorate the wall.
Consider using colors that represent summertime.

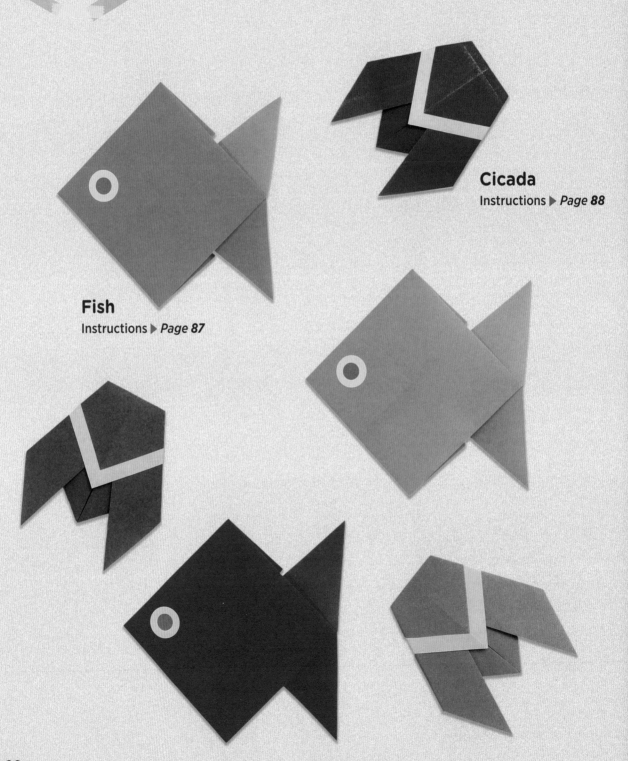

Cicada

Instructions ▶ *Page 88*

Fish

Instructions ▶ *Page 87*

Method 56

Challenge
▶ *Page 86*

Paper Size: 6 x 6 in (15 x 15 cm) square origami paper

Fish

To avoid unnecessary creases in the finished piece, steps ① and ② include a method for installing subtle landmarks. Take a little extra time to work carefully while making the pinch marks.

1 Curl the paper to match the top and bottom edges and make only a pinch mark on both sides (green reference marks) to indicate the horizontal center. Then, fold the top and bottom edges to these marks, crease, and unfold.

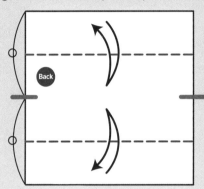

2 Repeat the actions of step ① from side to side to mark the vertical center. Then, fold the left and right edges to these marks, crease, and unfold.

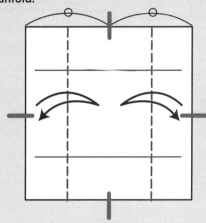

3 Flap A: valley fold between the pinch marks. Flap B: mountain fold between the pinch marks. Unfold, and then cut as indicated.

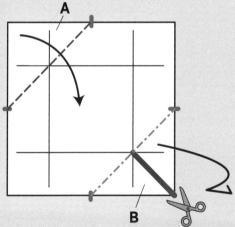

4 Fold along the existing creases to collapse the paper. Refer to the diagram for step ⑤ before folding.

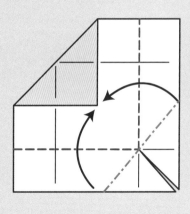

5 Make valley folds to finish the shape.

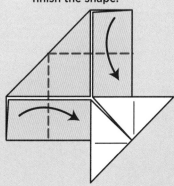

6 Flip it over and rotate to change the orientation.

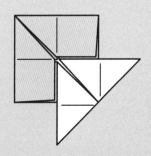

Turn over

Rotate

7 Finished. Draw or use stickers to indicate the eyes.

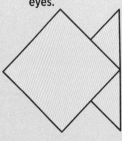

Paper Size: 6 x 6 in (15 x 15 cm) square origami paper

Cicada

In step 4, open the paper to the left and right to form the wings. If they are not perfectly symmetrical, it won't look quite right when finished. This piece has many layers, and you'll notice the thickness when holding the finished product.

① Fold the paper in half corner to corner.

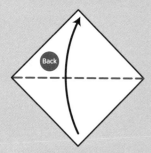

② Crease and unfold.

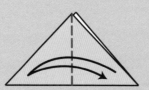

③ Fold to align the ☆ edges with the ★ crease.

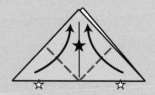

④ Pay attention to the indicated crease positions and valley fold the uppermost flaps on the left and right sides.

Zoom in

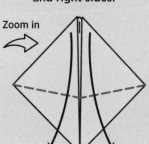

⑤ Pay attention to the indicated crease position and valley fold only the top layer.

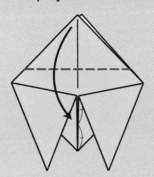

⑥ Make a valley fold slightly above the fold made in step ⑤.

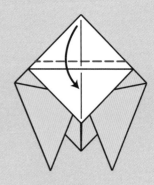

⑦ Flip it over.

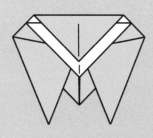

Turn over

⑧ Fold to align the ☆ edges with the ★ crease.

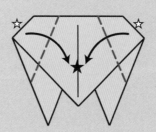

⑨ Flip it over.

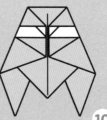

⑩ Finished.

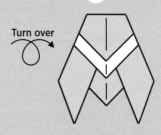

Turn over

Challenge 57

Star Festival Night (Tanabata)

Gather with others and write your wishes on strips of paper, then decorate the wall. Create your pieces with heartfelt wishes to make your dreams come true.

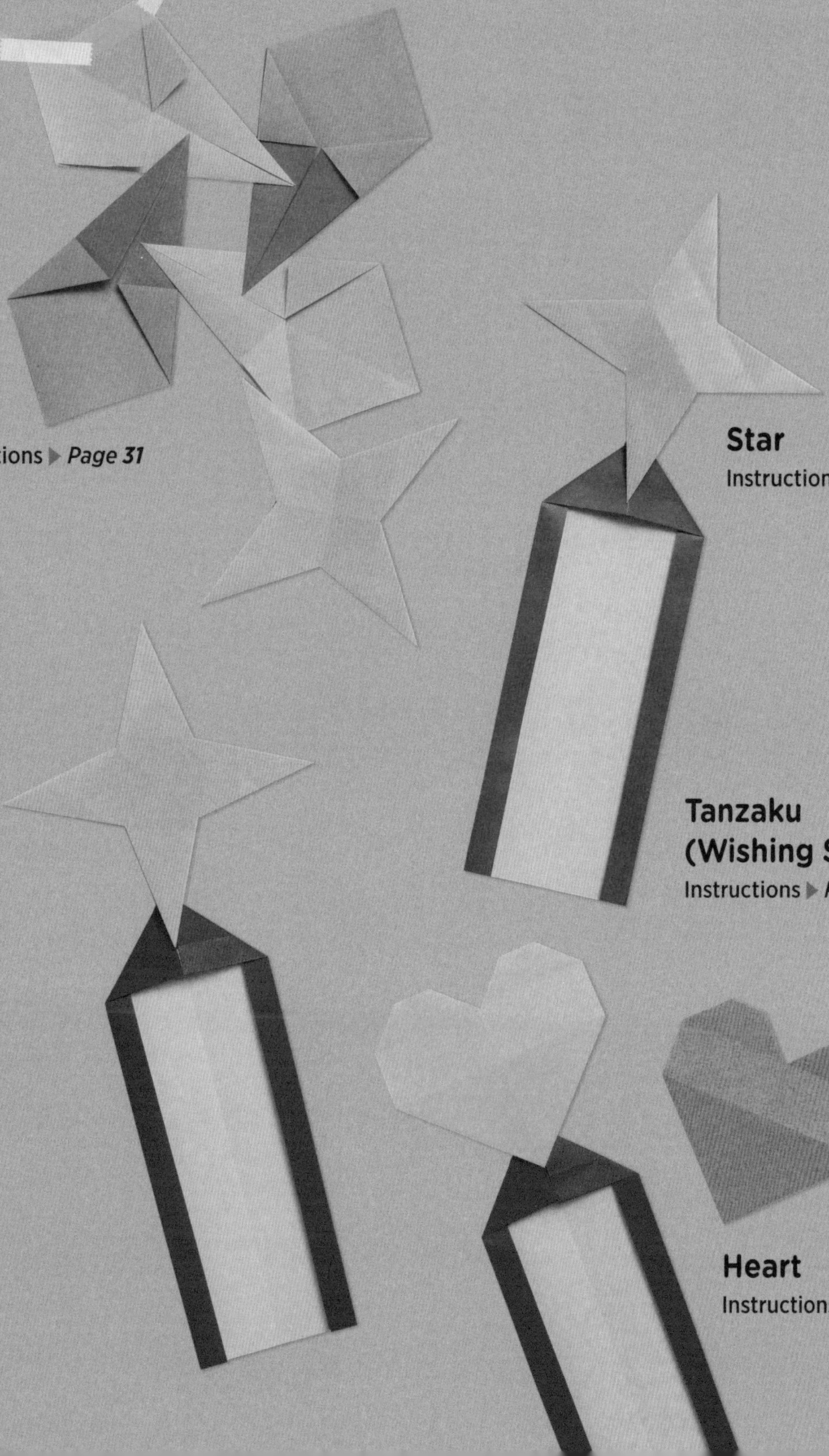

Instructions ▶ *Page 31*

Star
Instructions ▶ *Page 91*

**Tanzaku
(Wishing Strips)**
Instructions ▶ *Page 90*

Heart
Instructions ▶ *Page 91*

Challenge 58

Love

Why not express your feelings in origami form for a birthday or to commemorate a special occasion?

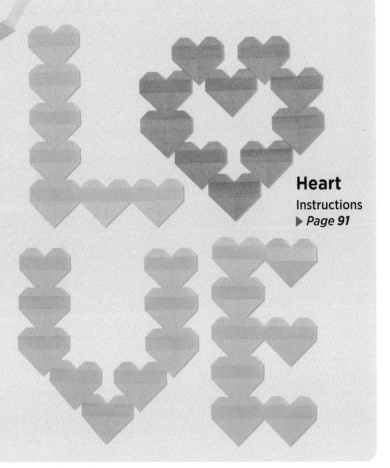

Heart
Instructions
▶ *Page 91*

Instructions

Method 57

Paper Size: Halve 6 x 6 in (15 x 15 cm) origami paper to get a 3 x 6 in (7.5 x 15 cm) rectangle.

Tanzaku (Wishing Strips)

Make many in various colors and write your wishes on them.

Challenge
▶ *Page 89*

1. Crease and unfold.

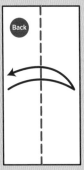

2. Make creases and unfold.

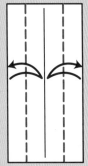

3. Fold the left and right edges to align with the creases made in step 2.

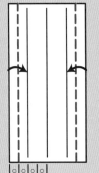

4. Fold in the top corners.

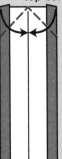

5. Finished.

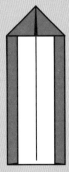

Method 57

Paper Size: Cut a 6 x 6 in (15 x 25 cm) piece of origami paper into quarters, resulting in 3 x 3 in (7.5 x 7.5 cm) squares.

Star

Challenge
▶ *Page 89*

You can also make a large star with the original 6 × 6 inch (15 × 15 cm) size paper.

1 Make creases and unfold.

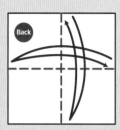

2 Make creases and unfold.

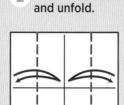

3 Make creases and unfold.

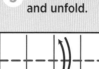

4 Make cuts along the creases.

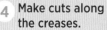
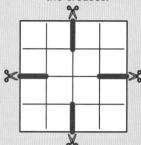

5 Fold the 8 flaps to overlap as indicated.

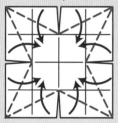

6 Flip it over.

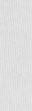
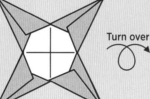

Turn over

7 Finished.

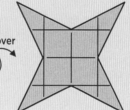

Method 50, 57, 58

Paper Size: Cut a 6 x 6 in (15 x 25 cm) piece of origami paper into quarters, resulting in 3 x 3 in (7.5 x 7.5 cm) squares.

Heart

Challenge
▶ *Page 72, 89, 90*

Matching the left and right sides at step 5 is the key to a neat finish!

1 Make creases and unfold.

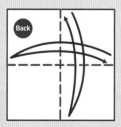

2 Make a crease and unfold.

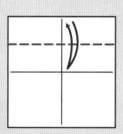

3 Cut along the crease.

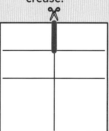

4 Fold the 4 top corners.

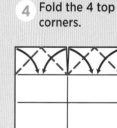

5 Fold in the bottom corners.

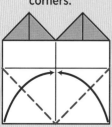

6 Fold the top 2 corners carefully.

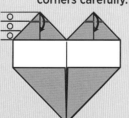

7 Flip it over.

8 Finished.

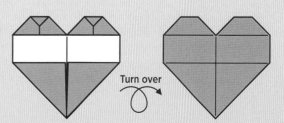

Turn over

Hydrangea

Snails ×2

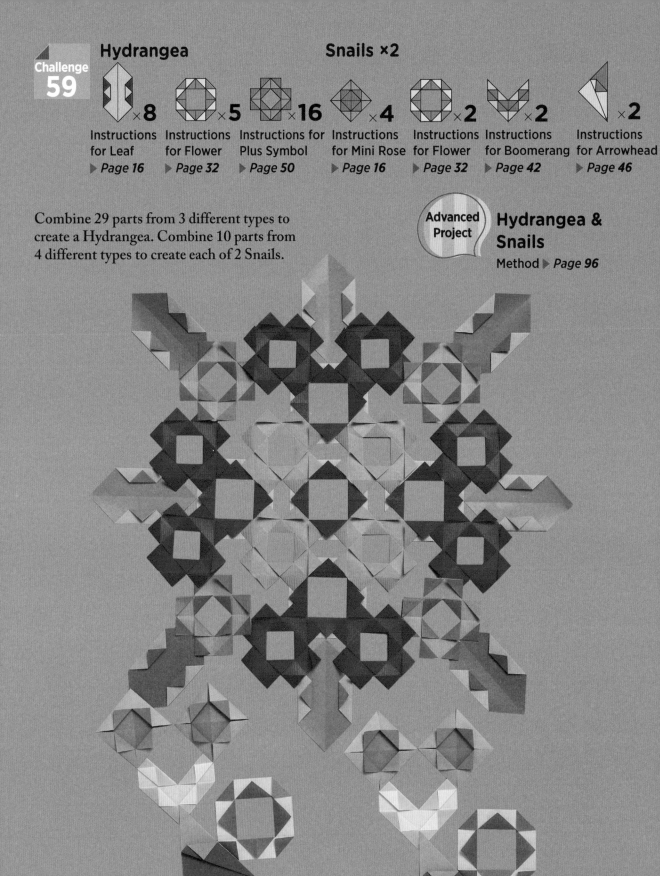

×8
Instructions for Leaf
▶ *Page 16*

×5
Instructions for Flower
▶ *Page 32*

×16
Instructions for Plus Symbol
▶ *Page 50*

×4
Instructions for Mini Rose
▶ *Page 16*

×2
Instructions for Flower
▶ *Page 32*

×2
Instructions for Boomerang
▶ *Page 42*

×2
Instructions for Arrowhead
▶ *Page 46*

Combine 29 parts from 3 different types to create a Hydrangea. Combine 10 parts from 4 different types to create each of 2 Snails.

Advanced Project

Hydrangea & Snails

Method ▶ *Page 96*

Challenge 60

Carp Streamer

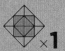 ×1
Instructions
for Mini Rose
▶ *Page 16*

 ×11
Instructions
for Drum
▶ *Page 50*

 ×5
Instructions
for Trapezoid
▶ *Page 62*

Helmet

 ×7
Instructions
for Mount Fuji
▶ *Page 20*

 ×2
Instructions
for Spearhead
▶ *Page 28*

Combine 17 parts from 3 different types to create a Carp Streamer. Combine 9 parts from 2 different types to create a Samurai Helmet.

Advanced Project

Carp Streamer & Samurai Helmet

Method ▶ *Page 98*

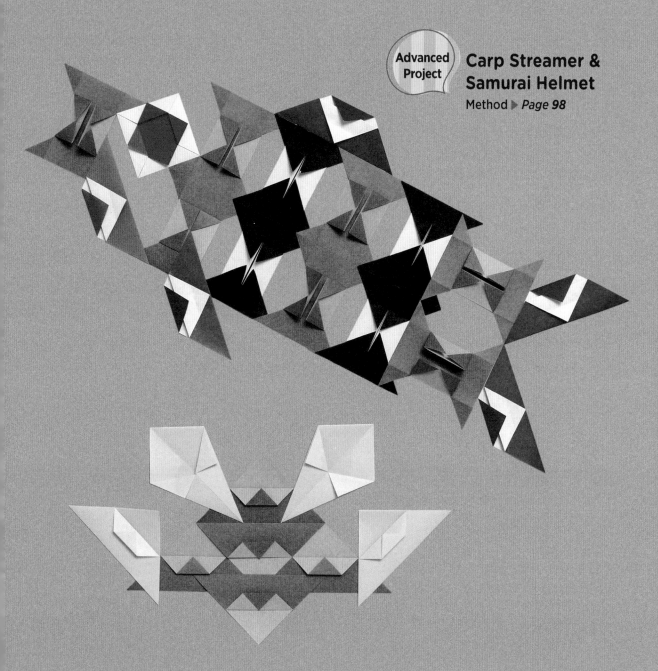

×**7**

Instructions
for Spearhead
▶ *Page 28*

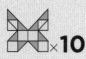×**10**

Instructions
for Butterfly
▶ *Page 36*

Combine 17 parts from 2 different types to
create the Sparkling Dance.

Advanced
Project

Sparkling Dance
Method ▶ *Page 100*

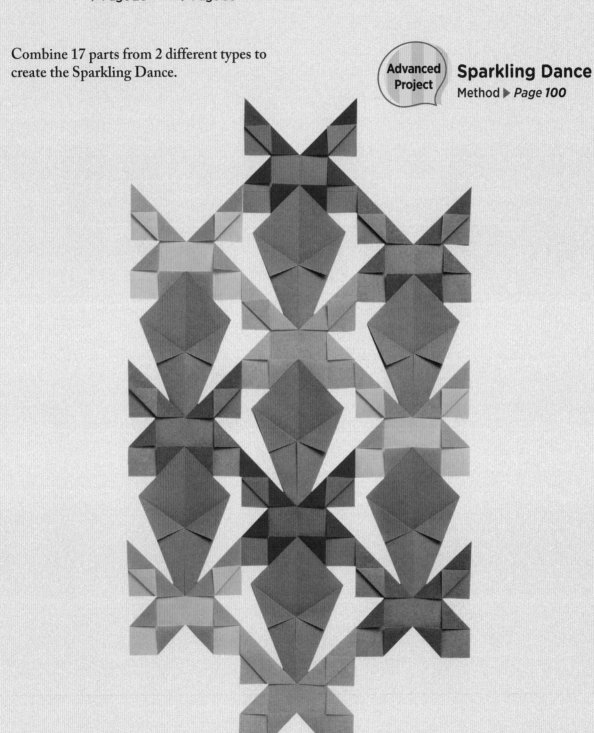

×**2**
Instructions
for Mini Rose
▶ *Page 16*

×**2**
Instructions
for Diamond
▶ *Page 20*

×**3**
Instructions
for M Shape
▶ *Page 42*

×**2**
Instructions
for Necktie
▶ *Page 54*

×**4**
Instructions
for Trapezoid
▶ *Page 62*

Combine 13 parts from 5 different types to create the Demon.

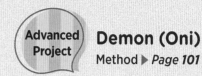

Advanced Project

Demon (Oni)
Method ▶ *Page 101*

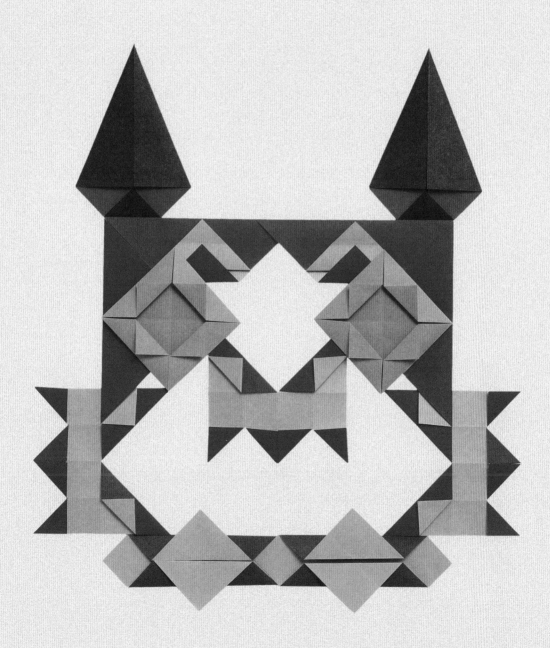

Method **59**

Hydrangea

×**8**
Instructions for Leaf ▶ *Page 16*

×**5**
Instructions for Flower ▶ *Page 32*

×**16**
Instructions for Plus Symbol ▶ *Page 50*

Snails ×2

×**4**
Instructions for Mini Rose ▶ *Page 16*

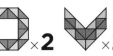×**2**
Instructions for Flower ▶ *Page 32*

×**2**
Instructions for Boomerang ▶ *Page 42*

×**2**
Instructions for Arrowhead ▶ *Page 46*

Advanced Project

Hydrangea and Snails
Challenge ▶ *Page 92*

1 Align the shapes as indicated. Superimpose 4 Plus Symbol parts on the Flower part and adhere them together.

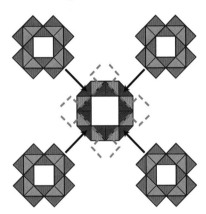

2 Building on the shape made in step 1, attach 4 Flower parts, aligning them with the reference lines. The Flower parts are superimposed by the Plus Symbol parts from step 1.

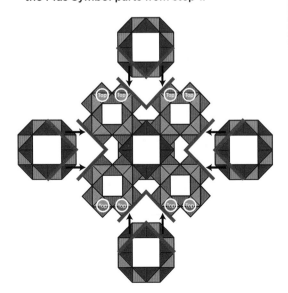

3 Align the shapes as indicated. Superimpose 8 Plus Symbol parts on the Flower parts from step 2 and adhere them together.

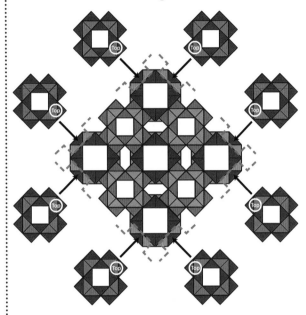

4 Use the blue-square part as a reference. Attach 4 Plus Symbol parts, aligning them with the reference lines. The 4 Plus Symbol parts are superimposed by the 8 Plus Symbol parts from step 3.

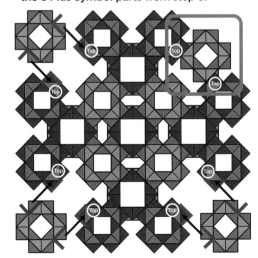

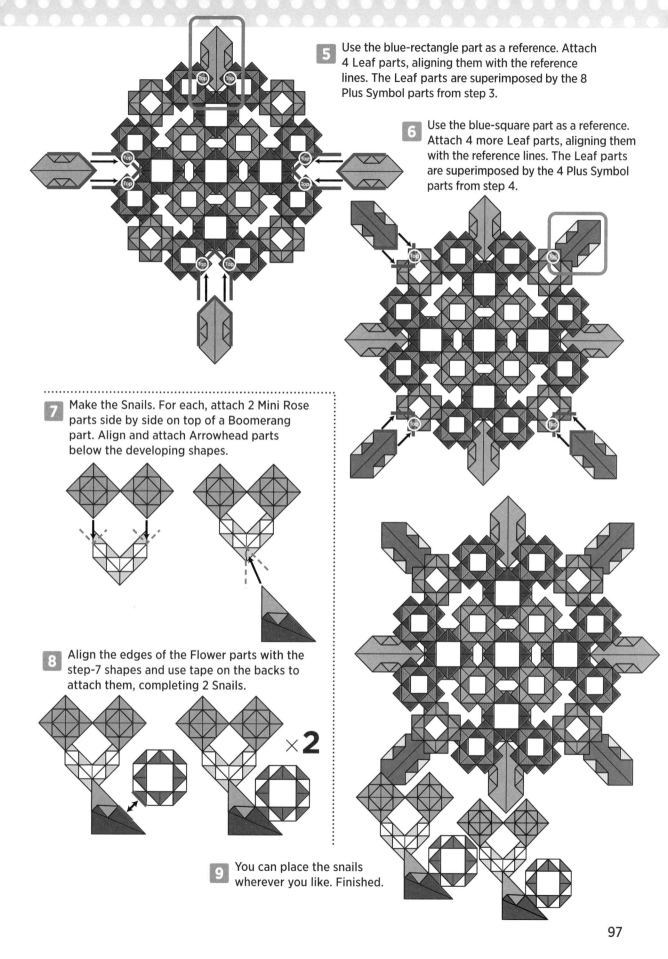

5 Use the blue-rectangle part as a reference. Attach 4 Leaf parts, aligning them with the reference lines. The Leaf parts are superimposed by the 8 Plus Symbol parts from step 3.

6 Use the blue-square part as a reference. Attach 4 more Leaf parts, aligning them with the reference lines. The Leaf parts are superimposed by the 4 Plus Symbol parts from step 4.

7 Make the Snails. For each, attach 2 Mini Rose parts side by side on top of a Boomerang part. Align and attach Arrowhead parts below the developing shapes.

8 Align the edges of the Flower parts with the step-7 shapes and use tape on the backs to attach them, completing 2 Snails.

×**2**

9 You can place the snails wherever you like. Finished.

Method 60

Carp Streamer

×1
Instructions for Mini Rose
▶ *Page 16*

×11
Instructions for Drum
▶ *Page 50*

×5
Instructions for Trapezoid
▶ *Page 62*

Helmet

×7
Instructions for Mount Fuji
▶ *Page 20*

×2
Instructions for Spearhead
▶ *Page 28*

Advanced Project

Carp Streamer & Samurai Helmet

Challenge ▶ *Page 93*

1 Align the edges of the Drum parts as indicated by the reference lines. Use tape on the back to adhere them together. Make 4 sets.

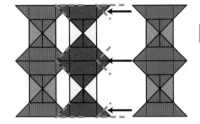

2 Align the shapes as indicated by the blue dashed lines. Adhere the 4 sets made in step 1 horizontally.

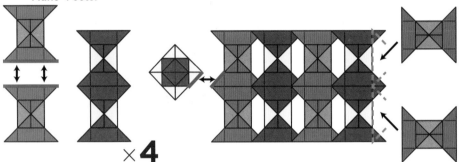

×**4**

3 Align the shapes as indicated by the blue dashed lines. Adhere 2 Drum parts superimposed on the step-2 assembly. Attach the Mini Rose part (the eye). Align the edges as indicated, and use tape on the back to adhere it.

4 Attach 5 Trapezoid parts to the step-3 assembly, paying attention to how they are aligned and attached.

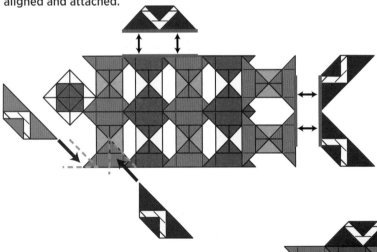

5 For the mouth, align the edges of the Drum part as indicated, and use tape on the back to adhere it. The Drum part will be superimposed by the step-4 assembly.

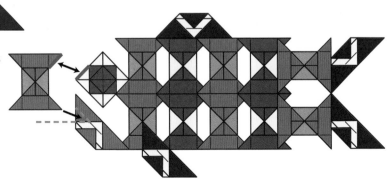

6 The Carp Streamer is finished.

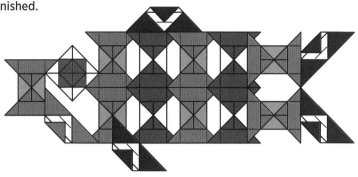

7 Make the Samurai Helmet. Align the edges of 4 Mount Fuji parts, alternating their orientation, and use tape on the back to adhere them together.

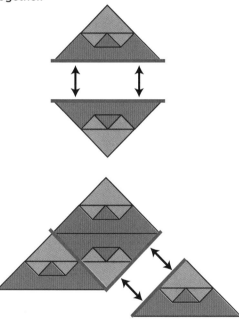

8 Align a superimposed Mount Fuji part with the step-7 assembly and adhere it.

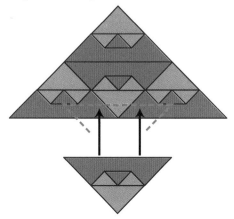

9 Add to the step-8 assembly by attaching 2 Spearhead parts and 2 Mount Fuji parts, all superimposed, ensuring that they are aligned as indicated.

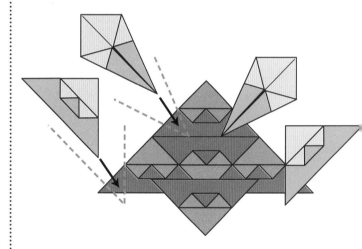

10 The Samurai Helmet is completed.

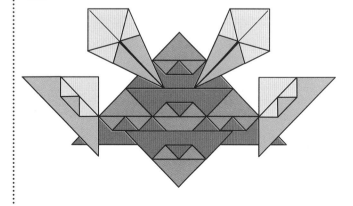

Method 61

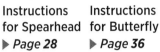

×**7**

Instructions for Spearhead ▶ Page 28

×**10**

Instructions for Butterfly ▶ Page 36

Advanced Project

Sparkling Dance

Challenge ▶ Page 94

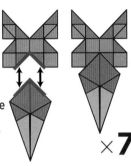

1 Align the edges of the Butterfly and Spearhead parts as indicated, and use tape on the back to adhere them together. Make 7 sets of the same.

×**7**

2 Align the edges of 3 of the sets made in step 1 as indicated, and use tape on the back to adhere them together. Repeat the same with another 3 sets.

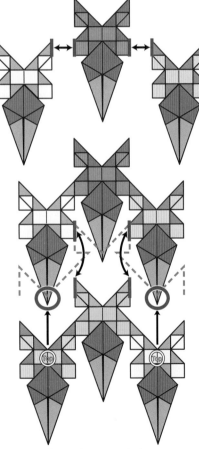

3 Adhere the step-2 shapes together, paying attention to the vertical alignment.

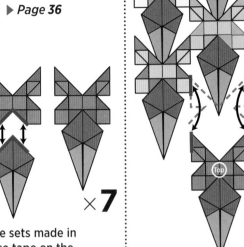

4 Align the edges of the remaining set made in step 1 as indicated by the blue dashed line, and use tape on the back to adhere them together.

5 Align the edges of 3 Butterfly parts as indicated, and use tape on the back to adhere them together.

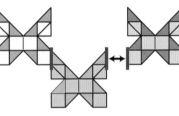

6 Align the shape made in step 5 as indicated by the reference lines, and adhere it using tape on the back.

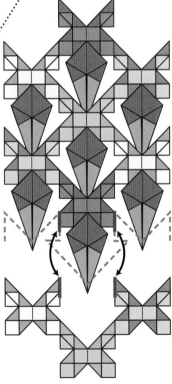

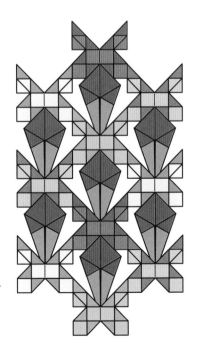

7 Finished.

Method 62

Advanced Project

Demon (Oni)

Challenge ▶ *Page 95*

×2 Instructions for Mini Rose ▶ *Page 16*

×2 Instructions for Diamond ▶ *Page 20*

×3 Instructions for M Shape ▶ *Page 42*

×2 Instructions for Necktie ▶ *Page 54*

×4 Instructions for Trapezoid ▶ *Page 62*

1 Align the edges of the Diamond and Trapezoid parts as indicated, and use tape on the back to adhere them together.

2 Attach the Mini Rose part (the eye) on top of the shape made in step 1.

3 Attach the M Shape part on top of the shape made in step 2, so that the shape from step 2 is on top.

4 Align the edge of the step-3 assembly and the Necktie part as indicated, and use tape on the back to adhere them together.

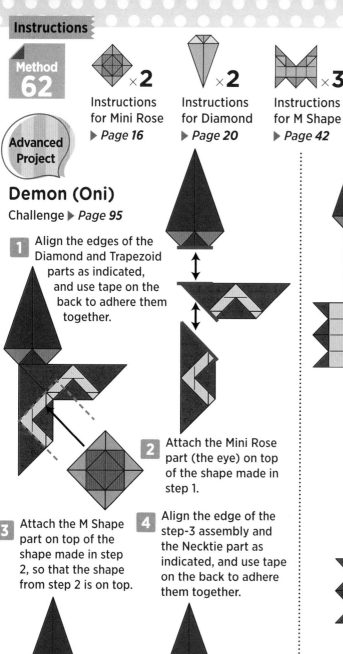

5 Following the same steps from 1 to 4, create the right side of the face in mirror image.

Attach the left and right sides of the face, ensuring the right side is on top.

6 Attach the M Shape part to make the nose.

7 Finished.

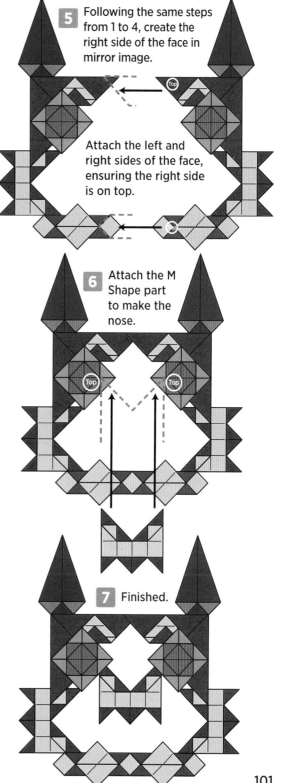

101

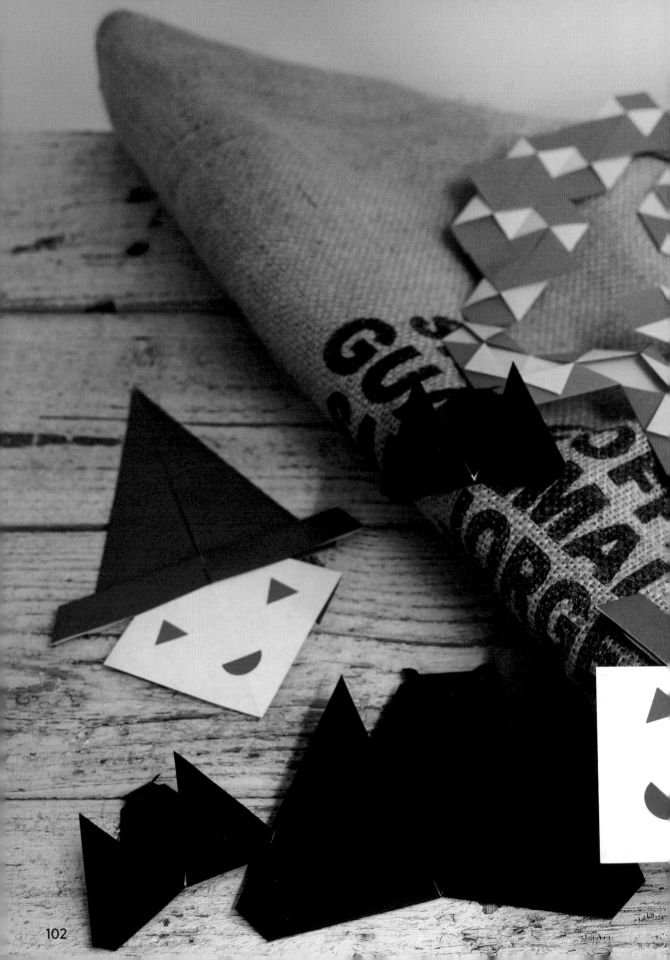

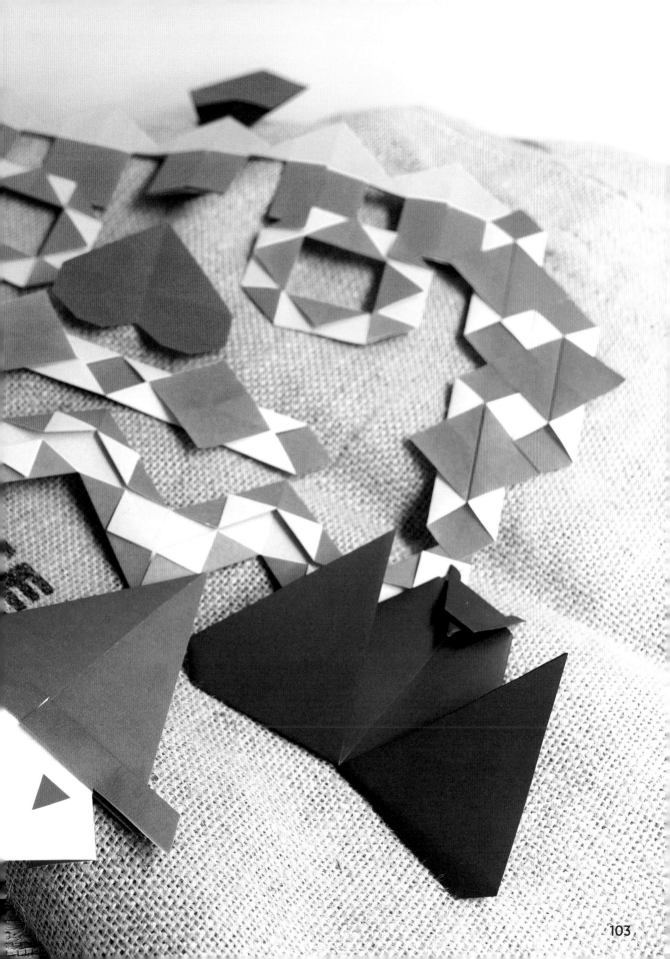

Challenge 63

Maple Leaves, Acorns & Mushrooms

Create autumn colors and shapes by hand to decorate the wall. These also look lovely on colored paper or postcards.

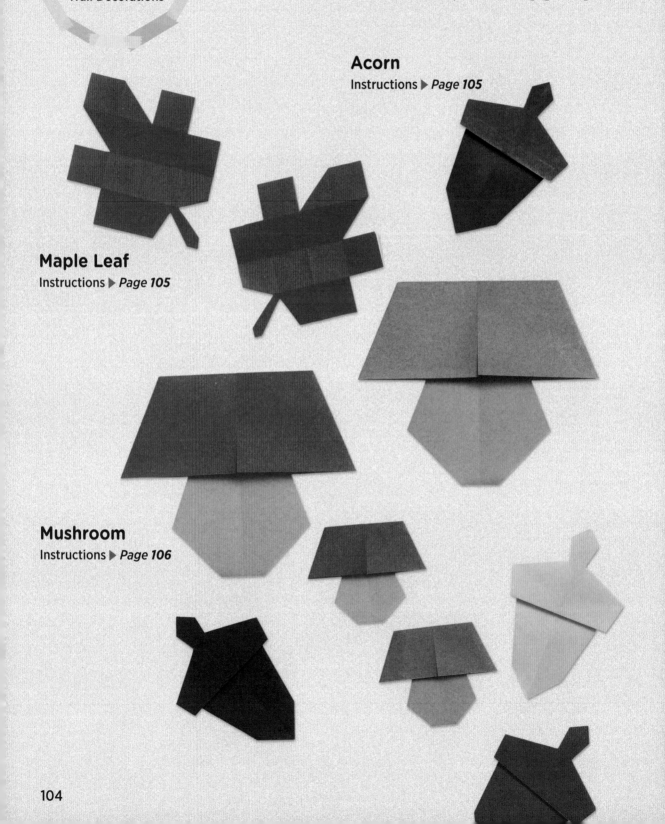

Acorn
Instructions ▶ *Page 105*

Maple Leaf
Instructions ▶ *Page 105*

Mushroom
Instructions ▶ *Page 106*

Method 63

Paper Size: Cut a 6 x 6 in (15 x 25 cm) piece of origami paper into quarters, resulting in 3 x 3 in (7.5 x 7.5 cm) squares.

Maple Leaf

Challenge
▶ *Page 104*

Use only the necessary parts of the many creases to create the shape.

1 Make creases and unfold.

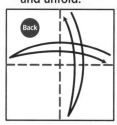

2 Make creases and unfold.

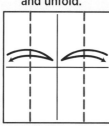

3 Make creases and unfold. Once done, rotate to change the orientation.

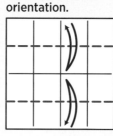

4 Make cuts along the creases.

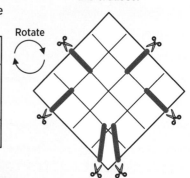

5 Fold 8 flaps as indicated.

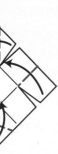

6 Flip it over.

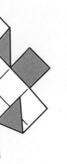

7 Finished.

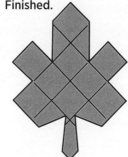

Method 63

Paper Size: Cut a 6 x 6 in (15 x 25 cm) piece of origami paper into quarters, resulting in 3 x 3 in (7.5 x 7.5 cm) squares.

Acorn

Challenge
▶ *Page 104*

Creating this piece symmetrically is important. Make many of them.

1 Fold the paper in half corner to corner.

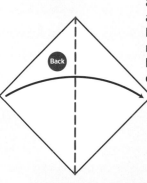

2 On the right side, pay attention to the position and valley fold through both layers and unfold. At the top, make a cut through both layers. Once done, open the entire piece.

3 Use the cuts to fold flaps on the left and right sides.

4 Use the creases from step 2 to fold the left and right sides.

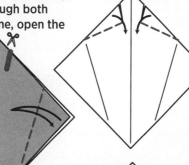

5 Pleat by installing adjacent horizontal mountain and valley folds.

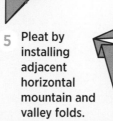

6 Flip it over.

7 Finished.

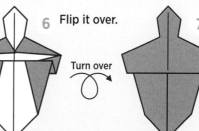

Method
63

Challenge
▶ *Page 104*

Paper Size: Cut a 6 x 6 in (15 x 25 cm) piece of origami paper into quarters, resulting in 3 x 3 in (7.5 x 7.5 cm) squares.

Mushroom

After completing the piece, if the folded paper on the back starts to lift, use double-sided tape to secure it.

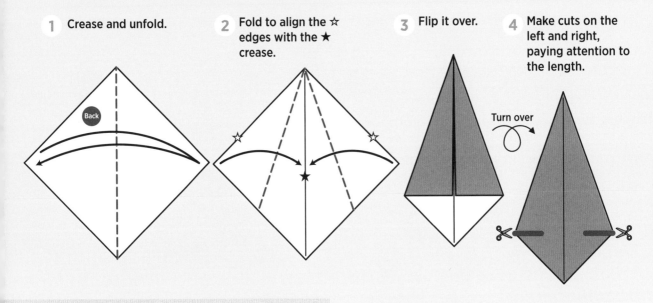

1 Crease and unfold.

2 Fold to align the ☆ edges with the ★ crease.

3 Flip it over.

4 Make cuts on the left and right, paying attention to the length.

Turn over

You can also use Maple Leaves to create an autumn wreath.

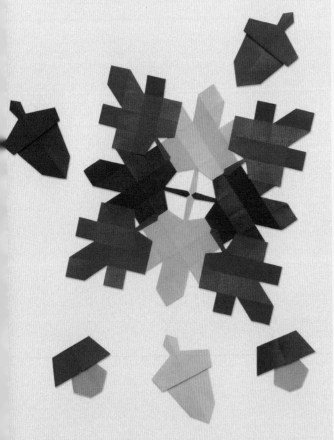

5 Use the cuts to fold the left and right flaps. Fold up a small portion of the bottom corner.

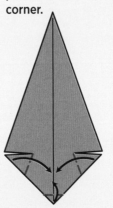

6 Valley fold the entire piece so that the pointed top corner is slightly above the bottom edge.

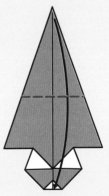

7 Flip it over.

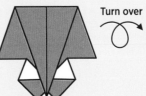

Turn over

8 Finished.

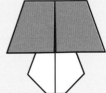

Witch & Bat

Challenge 64

What kind of face will you draw on the witch? Try making bats in different sizes.

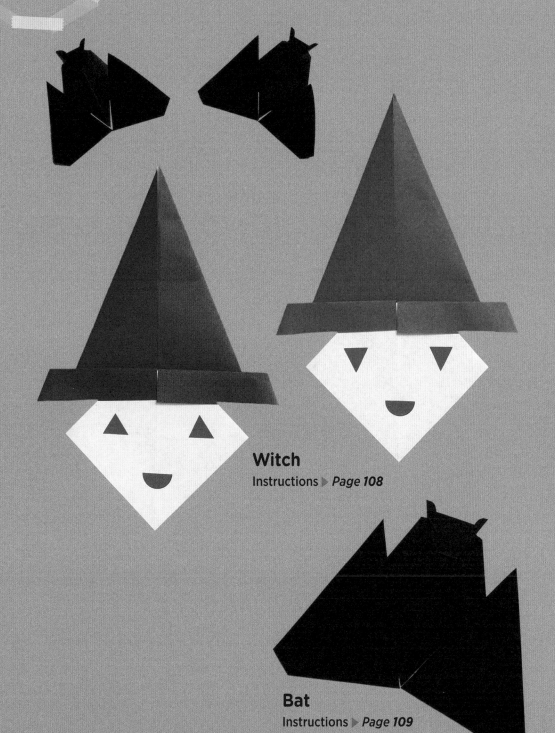

Witch
Instructions ▸ *Page 108*

Bat
Instructions ▸ *Page 109*

Method 64

Challenge
▶ Page 107

Paper Size: 6 x 6 in (15 x 15 cm) square origami paper

Witch

The length of the cuts in step 4 will affect the area and shape of the folded parts in step 5, thus changing the face shape. Be careful to make cuts of the same length on both sides.

1 Crease and unfold.

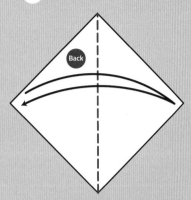

2 Fold to align the ☆ edges with the ★ crease.

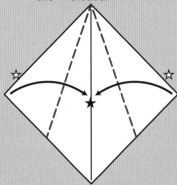

3 Flip it over.

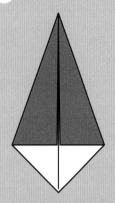

4 Make cuts on the left and right, paying attention to the length.

Turn over

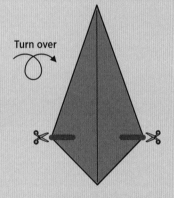

5 Use the cuts to fold the left and right flaps.

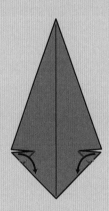

6 Valley fold the entire piece to bring the top pointed corner down.

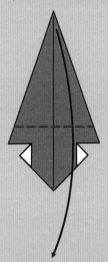

7 Valley fold just above the green reference line to bring the pointed corner back up.

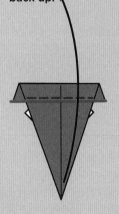

8 Flip it over.

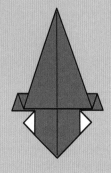

9 Finished. Draw on the face.

Turn over

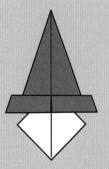

Method 64

Challenge
▶ *Page 107*

Bat

In step 6, alternate mountain and valley folds to add detail to the face and add expression. You can make this piece in any size as long as the paper is square. Try making different sizes.

1 Crease and unfold.

2 Fold to align the ☆ edges with the ★ crease.

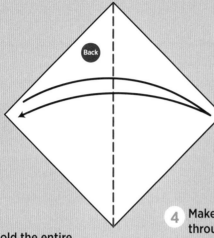

3 Fold the entire piece in half.

4 Make a curved cut through both layers for the ears. Once done, return the paper to the shape from step **3**.

5 Between the ends of the ear cuts, fold down the head carefully. Make a cut along the crease at the bottom, paying attention to the length.

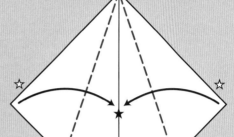

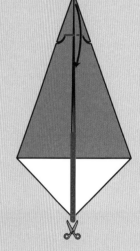

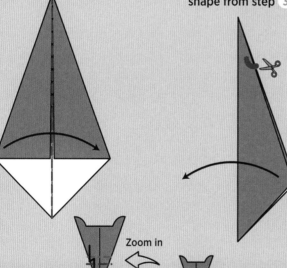

Zoom in

6 For the face, first make a mountain fold, then alternate with a valley fold. At the bottom, fold up the flaps and spread them to the sides.

7 Finished.

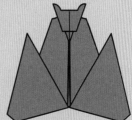

×5

Instructions for House
▶ *Page 24*

 ×1

Instructions for Spearhead
▶ *Page 28*

 ×2

Instructions for Flower
▶ *Page 32*

 ×4

Instructions for Boomerang
▶ *Page 42*

×8

Instructions for Necktie
▶ *Page 54*

 ×1

Instructions for Heart
▶ *Page 91*

Combine 21 parts from 6 different types to create the Halloween Jack-o'-Lantern. decoration.

Advanced Project

Halloween Jack-o'-Lantern
Instructions ▶ *Page 114*

Bat
Instructions ▶ *Page 109*

Witch
Instructions ▶ *Page 108*

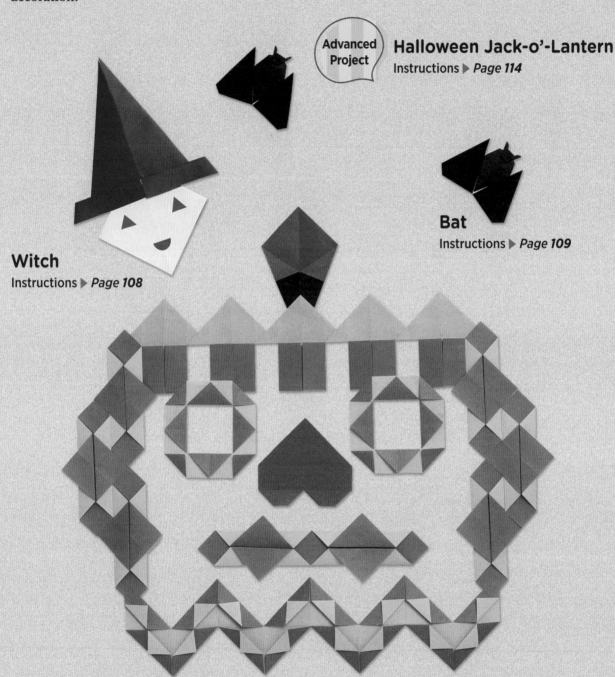

×3
Instructions
for Leaf
▶ *Page 16*

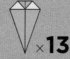 ×13
Instructions
for Diamond
▶ *Page 20*

 ×2
Instructions
for Flower
▶ *Page 32*

 ×1
Instructions
for Boomerang
▶ *Page 42*

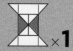 ×1
Instructions
for Drum
▶ *Page 50*

Combine 20 parts from 5 different types to create the Owl.

Advanced
Project

Owl
Method ▶ *Page 116*

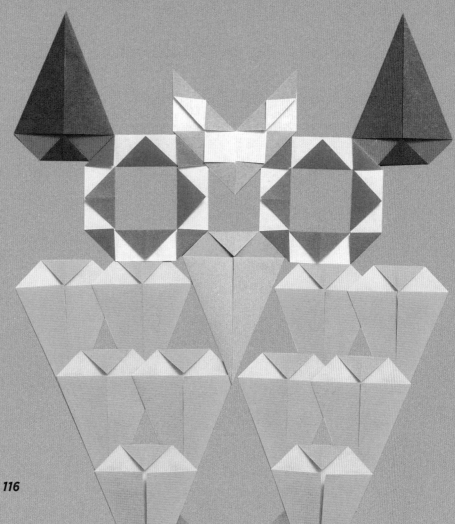

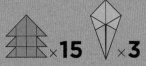 **×15**

 ×3

 ×3

×3

Instructions for Tree ▶ *Page 28*

Instructions for Spearhead ▶ *Page 28*

Instructions for Drum ▶ *Page 50*

Instructions for Star ▶ *Page 91*

Combine 24 parts from 4 different types and to make a Christmas Tree.

Advanced Project

Christmas Tree
Method ▶ *Page 118*

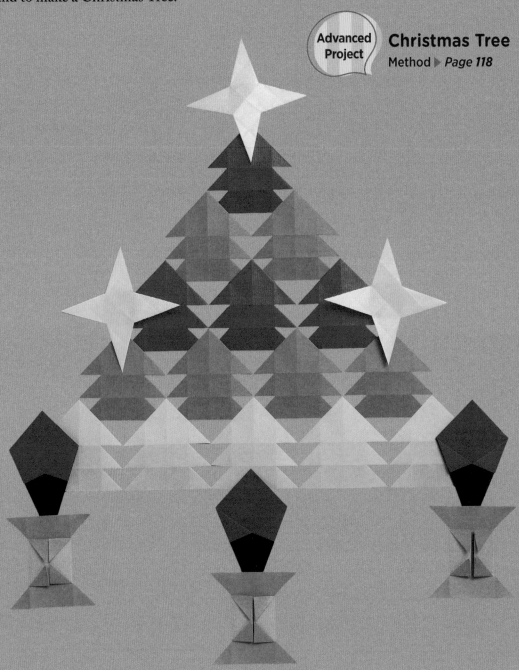

×**8**

Instructions
for Gem
▶ *Page 58*

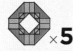×**5**

Instructions
for Prism
▶ *Page 62*

Combine 13 parts from 2
different types to make a
Hanging Decoration.

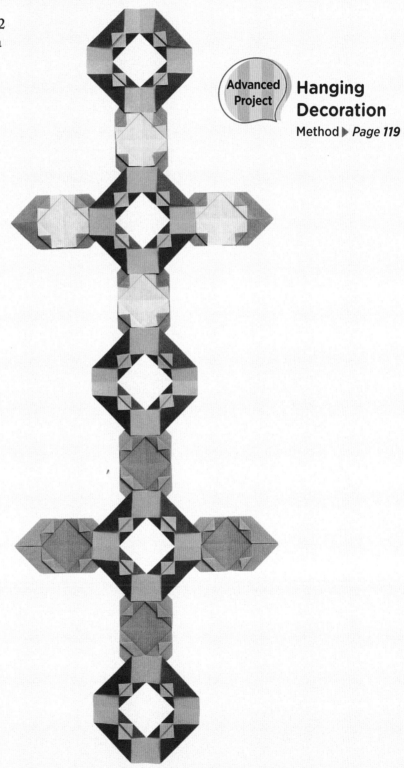

Advanced Project

Hanging Decoration

Method ▶ *Page 119*

Method 65

 ×**5**

Instructions
for House
▶ *Page 24*

 ×**1**

Instructions for
Spearhead
▶ *Page 28*

 ×**2**

Instructions
for Flower
▶ *Page 32*

 ×**4**

Instructions
for Boomerang
▶ *Page 42*

 ×**8**

Instructions
for Necktie
▶ *Page 54*

 ×**1**

Instructions
for Heart
▶ *Page 91*

Advanced Project

Halloween Jack-o'-Lantern
Challenge ▶ *Page 110*

1 Arrange 5 House parts horizontally and arrange them, aligning them as indicated. Pay attention to the relationships of the overlapping areas.

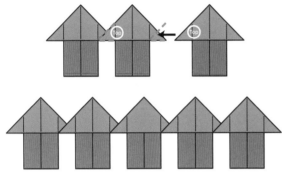

2 Attach the Spearhead part so the step-1 assembly superimposes. Align it to the reference line and adhere it.

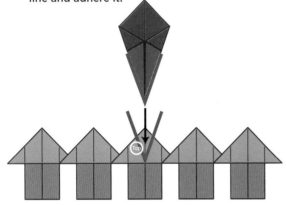

3 Align 4 Boomerang parts horizontally, match the edges as indicated, and use tape on the back to adhere them together.

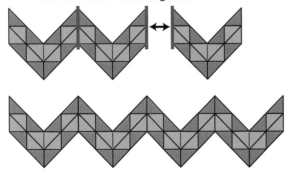

4 Match the edges of 3 Necktie parts, and use tape on the back to adhere them together. Also make a mirror-image shape using the same method.

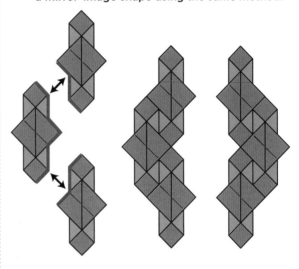

5 Align 2 Necktie parts as indicated, and adhere them with the right side superimposing.

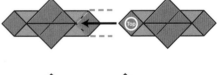

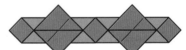

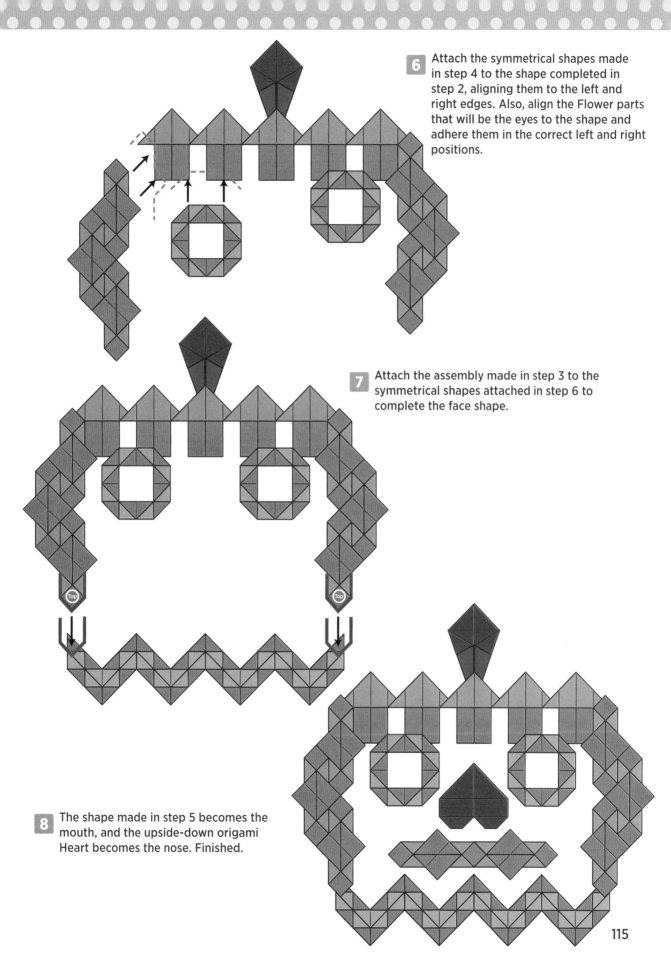

6 Attach the symmetrical shapes made in step 4 to the shape completed in step 2, aligning them to the left and right edges. Also, align the Flower parts that will be the eyes to the shape and adhere them in the correct left and right positions.

7 Attach the assembly made in step 3 to the symmetrical shapes attached in step 6 to complete the face shape.

8 The shape made in step 5 becomes the mouth, and the upside-down origami Heart becomes the nose. Finished.

Method 66

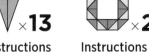

×**3**

Instructions for Leaf
▶ *Page 16*

×**13**

Instructions for Diamond
▶ *Page 20*

 ×**2**

Instructions for Flower
▶ *Page 32*

 ×**1**

Instructions for Boomerang
▶ *Page 42*

×**1**

Instructions for Drum
▶ *Page 50*

Advanced Project

Owl
Challenge ▶ *Page 111*

1 Make the Owl's face. Place the Flower parts that will become the eyes in the center. Align each part's edges and use tape on the back to adhere them together.

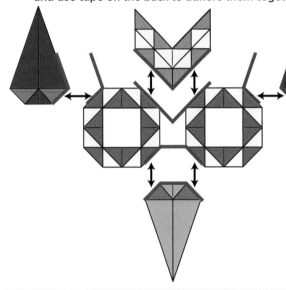

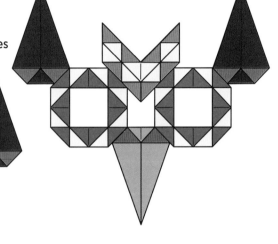

2 Make the wings. Align 2 Diamond parts and adhere them together. Make 4 sets of the same shape.

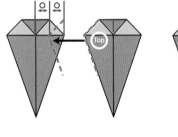

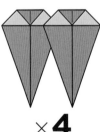

×**4**

3 Take 2 sets from step 2, align them with the diagonal line on the left edge, and adhere them together. Below that, align 1 more Diamond part with the diagonal line on the left edge and adhere it so that the final Diamond part superimposes the part it's attached to.

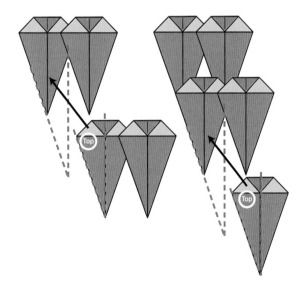

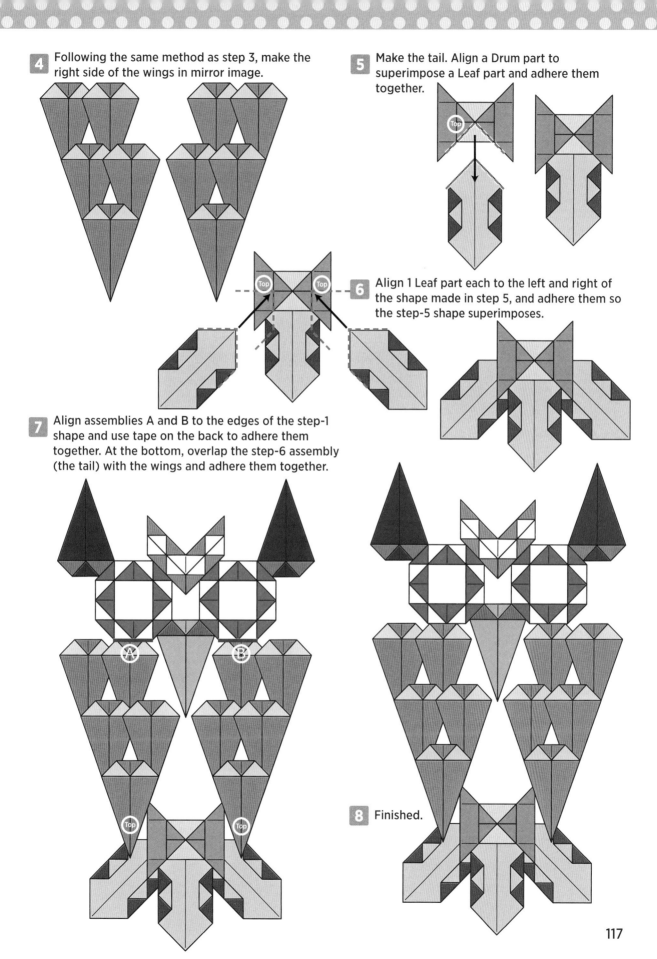

4 Following the same method as step 3, make the right side of the wings in mirror image.

5 Make the tail. Align a Drum part to superimpose a Leaf part and adhere them together.

6 Align 1 Leaf part each to the left and right of the shape made in step 5, and adhere them so the step-5 shape superimposes.

7 Align assemblies A and B to the edges of the step-1 shape and use tape on the back to adhere them together. At the bottom, overlap the step-6 assembly (the tail) with the wings and adhere them together.

8 Finished.

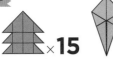

 ×**15**

Instructions for Tree
▶ *Page 28*

×**3**

Instructions for Spearhead
▶ *Page 28*

 ×**3**

Instructions for Drum
▶ *Page 50*

 ×**3**

Instructions for Star
▶ *Page 91*

Advanced Project

Christmas Tree

Challenge ▶ *Page 112*

1 Align a Drum part to superimpose a Spearhead part and adhere them together.

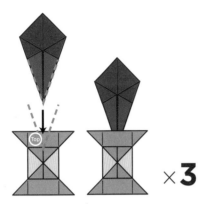

×**3**

2 Superimpose a Tree part with 2 others to form a pyramid shape. Align as shown and adhere them together.

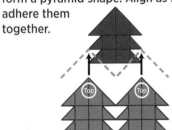

3 Below the step-2 shape, adhere more Tree parts in the same way, continuing the pyramid shape. Assemble 5 tiers using 15 parts.

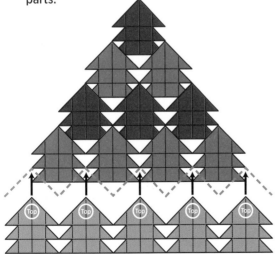

4 Align and adhere 3 Origami Stars superimposed on of the pyramid shape from step 3. Also, align and adhere the 3 sets made in step 1 as indicated.

5 Finished.

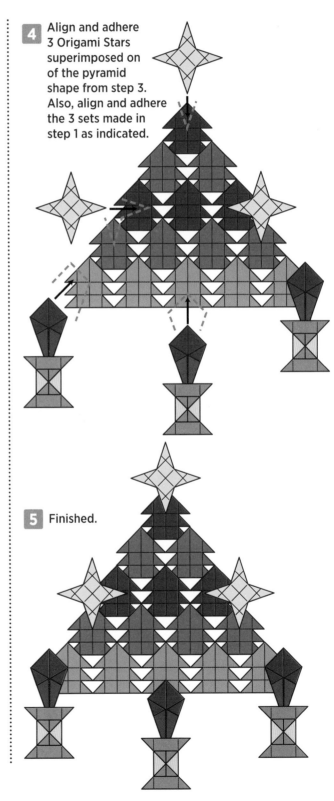

Method 68

 ×8
Instructions for Gem
▶ *Page 58*

 ×5
Instructions for Prism
▶ *Page 62*

Advanced Project

Hanging Ornament

Challenge ▶ *Page 113*

1 Using the pink-rectangle part as a reference, align 4 Gem parts around the Prism part with the Prism part superimposed, and adhere them as indicated. Make 2 sets of the same shape.

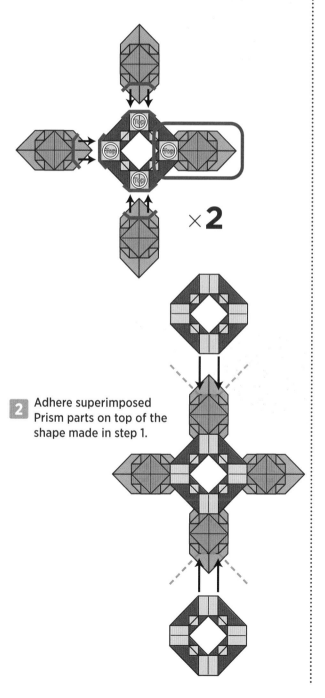

×2

2 Adhere superimposed Prism parts on top of the shape made in step 1.

3 Use the Prism parts to connect the shapes vertically. The ultimate length is up to you. Arrange to suit the atmosphere of the room. Finished.

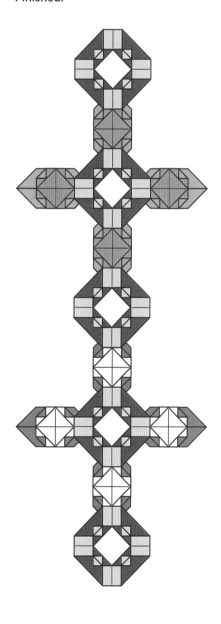

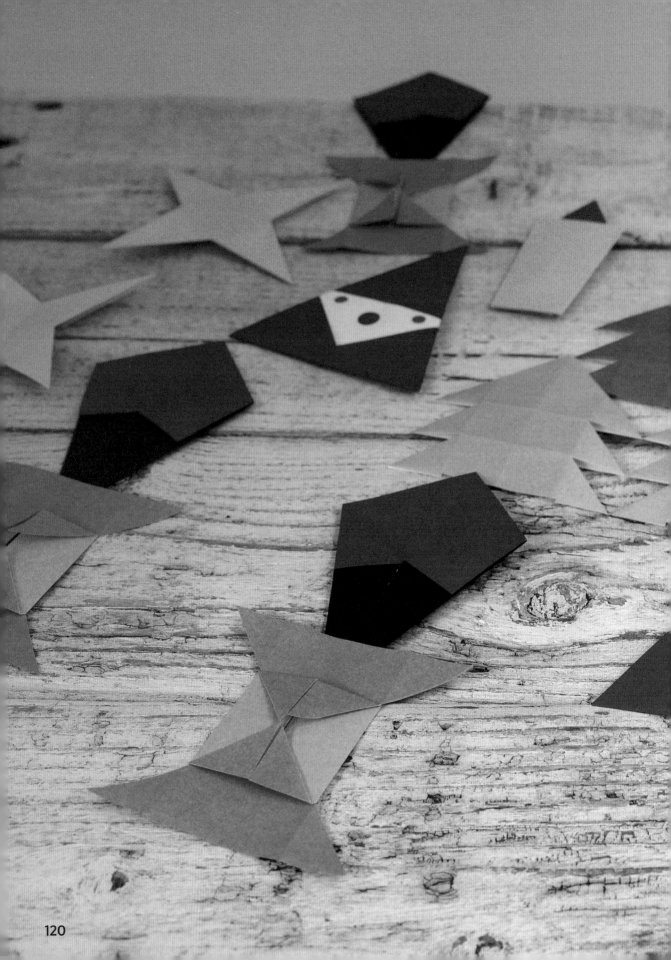

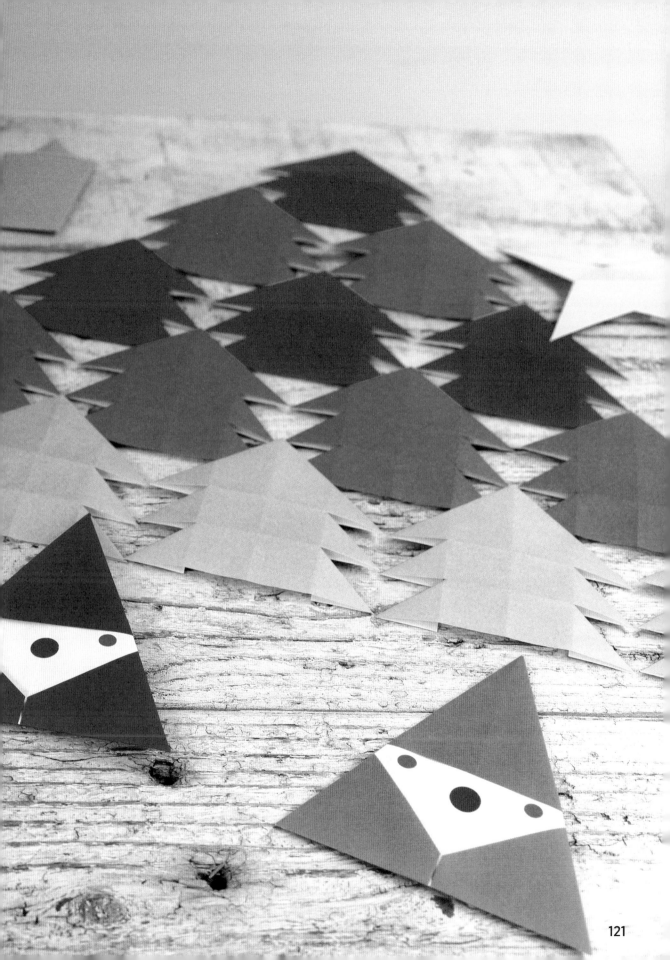

Challenge 69

Christmas Favorites

In addition to using these to decorate a wall, you can also use them as ornaments to hang on a Christmas tree.

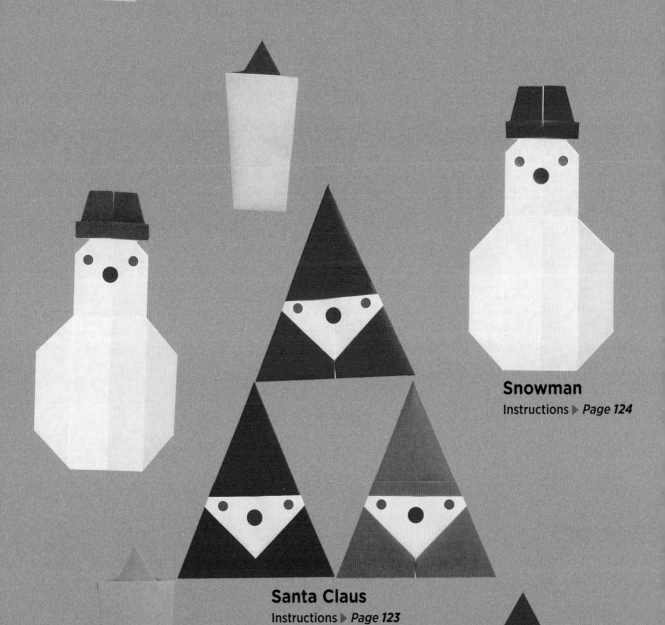

Snowman
Instructions ▶ *Page 124*

Santa Claus
Instructions ▶ *Page 123*

Candle
Instructions ▶ *Page 125*

Paper Size: 6 x 6 in (15 x 15 cm) square origami paper

Method
69

Challenge
▶ *Page 122*

Santa Claus

This Santa Claus wears a pointy hat and is finished as an isosceles triangle. You can also use this triangular silhouette to assemble a pyramid of jolly figures.

1 Crease and unfold.

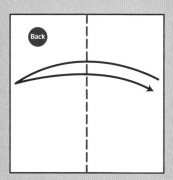

2 Fold both top corners in.

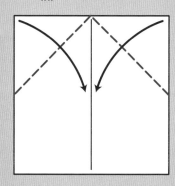

3 Fold to align the ☆ edges with the ★ crease.

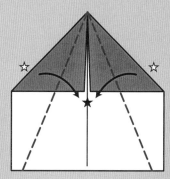

4 Valley fold a narrow strip from the bottom, paying attention to the position.

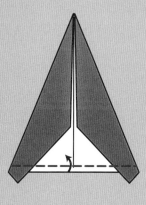

5 Flip it over.

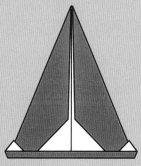

6 Fold the entire piece with a valley fold, bringing the pointed top corner down. Refer to the diagram for step **7** before you begin folding.

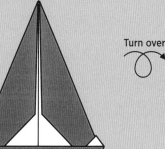

Turn over

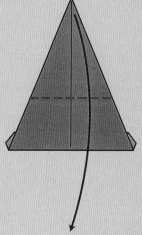

7 Fold the left and right sides along the edges of the triangular flap created in step **6**.

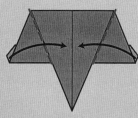

8 Flip it over and rotate it to change the orientation.

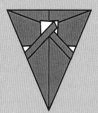

Turn over

Rotate

9 Finished.

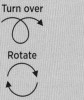
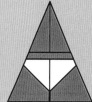

Paper Size: Cut a 6 x 6 in (15 x 25 cm) piece of origami paper in half to make a 6 x 3 in (15 x 7.5 cm) rectangle.

Snowman

Note that the length of the cuts in step 5 are different at the top and bottom. Carefully folding the corners will express the "roundness" of the snowman.

1 Crease and unfold.

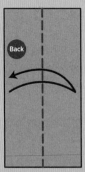

2 Crease and unfold.

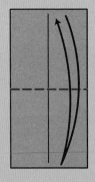

3 Make creases and unfold.

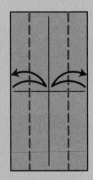

4 Crease and unfold.

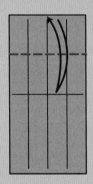

5 Make cuts along the creases. Note that the top cuts are slightly longer.

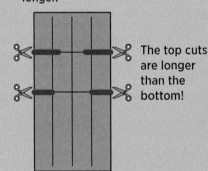

The top cuts are longer than the bottom!

6 Make valley folds.

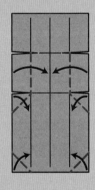

7 Make mountain folds on the left and right sides at the top.

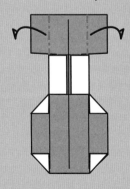

8 At the top, first make a mountain fold, then follow with a valley fold, forming a small pleat. Underneath, use the slightly longer cuts made in step 5 to fold the left and right corners of the head.

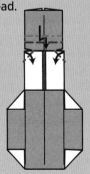

9 Taper the hat. Flip it over.

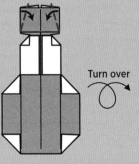

Turn over

10 Finished. Draw on a face.

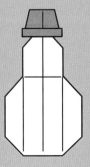

Method

69

Challenge
▶ *Page 122*

Paper Size: Cut a 6 x 6 in (15 x 25 cm) piece of origami paper in half to make a 6 x 3 in (15 x 7.5 cm) rectangle.

Candle

For this model, you can use double-sided origami paper that is colored on both sides, but make sure that the part that will become the flame has a warm color.

1 At the center of the top edge, divide the angle into 3 equal parts, and fold in the left corner.

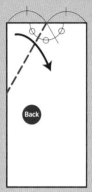

2 Following the same method as in step **1**, fold in the right corner.

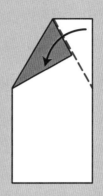

3 Flip it over.

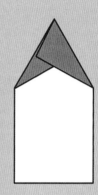

4 Fold up the bottom part. Refer to the diagram for step **5** before you begin folding. Once done, flip it over.

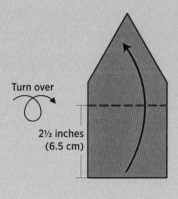

Turn over

2½ inches
(6.5 cm)

Zoom in

Turn over

5 Be mindful of the intended crease positions and fold both sides symmetrically.

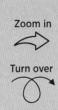

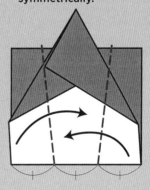

6 Flip it over.

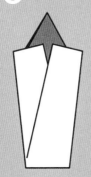

Turn over

7 Finished.

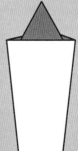

Peach Festival (Hina Matsuri)

To create beautiful origami compositions, it's essential to understand the characteristics of paper, use of the tools, and the folding methods and combination techniques. Familiarize yourself with these concepts thoroughly.

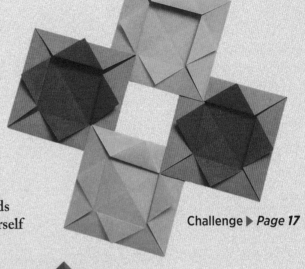

Challenge ▶ *Page 17*

Obina
Instructions ▶ *Page 127*

Mebina
Instructions ▶ *Page 127*

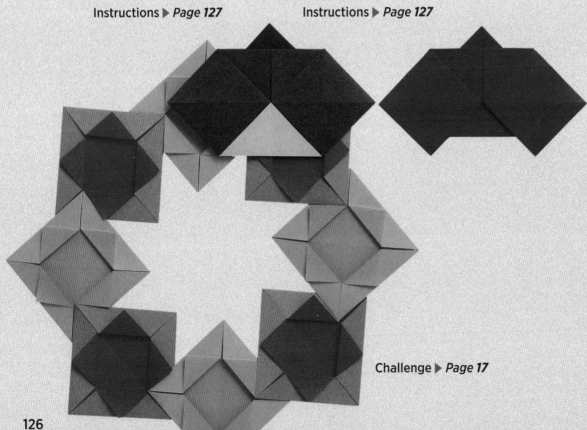

Challenge ▶ *Page 17*

Paper Size: 6 x 6 in (15 x 15 cm) square origami paper

Hina Dolls (Obina & Mebina)

Method **70**

Challenge
▶ *Page 126*

Steps 1 to 7 are the same for both Obina (the male doll, often representing the Emperor) and Mebina (the female doll, representing the Empress). Using paper with traditional Japanese patterns, like *chiyogami*, will enhance the doll-like characteristics.

1 Fold the paper in half corner to corner.

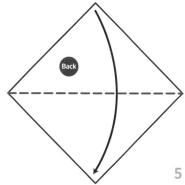

2 Crease and unfold.

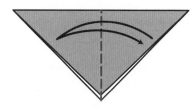

3 Fold to align the ☆ edges with the ★ crease.

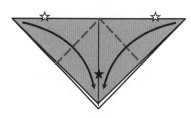

4 Fold up the bottom corners of the flaps folded in step 3.

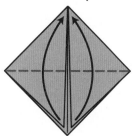

5 Insert your fingers into the pockets formed at step 2 to open up the paper.

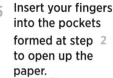

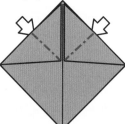

6 Step 5 in progress.

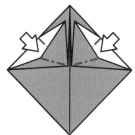

7 Install a mountain fold, followed by an adjacent valley fold, forming a narrow pleat.

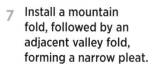

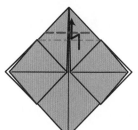

8 For Obina, fold up the top layer only.

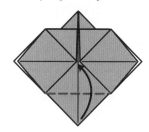

9 For Obina, perform a mountain fold on the lower sheet and tuck it behind.

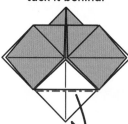

10 Obina is finished.

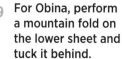

11 For Mebina, perform a mountain fold on both layers of the bottom part and tuck it behind.

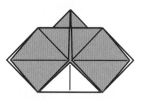

12 Mebina is finished.

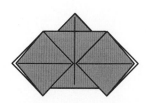

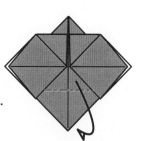

Afterword: The Baton Passed On

Since the publication of *Beautiful Cut Paper to Color Your Life* (Nagaoka Bookstore) in December of 2007, I have had many opportunities to present my work in numerous books. My creative activities have continued thanks to the efforts of publishers and the passionate support of the readers.

During this time, I met someone at a kirigami exhibition who was not only a fan of my books, but was also a creator in their own right, sharing with me how much they enjoyed handmade crafts. What I convey in my work is the kernel of creativity that develops into the enjoyment of handcrafting. To put it another way, the baton is passed on to others who incorporate handcrafting into their lives, assigning to the book a truly practical role.

Thank you, Yasuchika Hiruma-san and Mrs. Midori, for your wonderful creations.

Mayumi Ohara is a sculptor and graphic designer. In addition to editing and designing books, she creates handmade crafts. She began with kirigami and expanded her repertoire to include origami, beadwork, ceramics and flower arranging. She has written many books on origami, papercrafts and puzzles.

Professor Katsushi Yokoi is Vice Dean of the Department of Occupational Therapy at Morinomiya University of Medical Sciences in Osaka, Japan.

Medical Advisor: Katsushi Yokoi

Staff for the Japanese edition
Project Planning/Editing: Hideki Ohara
Photography: Keishi Shiraishi
Special thanks to Mikiko Yamaguchi for help with the photography
Book Design: Naoki Ogawa
Graphic Design/Layout: Masaru Yamazaki, Hideki Ohara

"Books to Span the East and West"

Tuttle Publishing was founded in 1832 in the small New England town of Rutland, Vermont [USA]. Our core values remain as strong today as they were then—to publish best-in-class books which bring people together one page at a time. In 1948, we established a publishing outpost in Japan—and Tuttle is now a leader in publishing English-language books about the arts, languages and cultures of Asia. The world has become a much smaller place today and Asia's economic and cultural influence has grown. Yet the need for meaningful dialogue and information about this diverse region has never been greater. Over the past seven decades, Tuttle has published thousands of books on subjects ranging from martial arts and paper crafts to language learning and literature—and our talented authors, illustrators, designers and photographers have won many prestigious award. We welcome you to explore the wealth of information available on Asia at **www.tuttlepublishing.com**.

Published by Tuttle Publishing, an imprint of Periplus Editions (HK) Ltd.

www.tuttlepublishing.com

978-4-8053-1895-9

No wo Kitaeru Block Origami
Copyright © 2019 Mayumi Ohara
English translation rights arranged with Seibundo Shinkosha Publishing Co., Ltd. through Japan UNI Agency, Inc., Tokyo

Printed in China   2411EP
28 27 26 25 24   10 9 8 7 6 5 4 3 2 1

TUTTLE PUBLISHING® is a registered trademark of Tuttle Publishing, a division of Periplus Editions (HK) Ltd.

Distributed by

North America, Latin America & Europe
Tuttle Publishing
364 Innovation Drive
North Clarendon,
VT 05759-9436 U.S.A.
Tel: (802) 773-8930
Fax: (802) 773-6993
info@tuttlepublishing.com
www.tuttlepublishing.com

Japan
Tuttle Publishing
Yaekari Building, 3rd Floor
5-4-12 Osaki
Shinagawa-ku
Tokyo 141-0032
Tel: (81) 3 5437-0171
Fax: (81) 3 5437-0755
sales@tuttle.co.jp
www.tuttle.co.jp

Asia Pacific
Berkeley Books Pte. Ltd.
3 Kallang Sector #04-01
Singapore 349278
Tel: (65) 6741-2178
Fax: (65) 6741-2179
inquiries@periplus.com.sg
www.tuttlepublishing.com